RECLAIMING MEMORIES

A Guide to Preventing and Navigating Dementia

Hope Ajagun

Copyright © 2024 Hope Ajagun

All rights reserved. No part of this book may be reproduced, or stored in a retrieval system, or transmitted in any form or by any means, electronic, mechanical, photocopying, recording, or otherwise, without express written permission of the publisher.

ISBN: 9798301060212

Cover design by: Art Painter
Printed in the United States of America

To those with health concerns and their loved ones

CONTENTS

Title Page

Copyright

Dedication

Introduction

Acknowledgments

Chapter 1: Understanding Dementia: A Biochemical Perspective	1
Chapter 2: Risk Factors and Prevention Strategies	7
Chapter 3: The Brain: A Marvel of Biochemistry	11
Chapter 4: Neurotransmitters: The Brain's Chemical Messengers	15
Chapter 5: Neurotransmitters and Cognitive Decline	19
Chapter 6: Energy Metabolism in the Brain	23
Chapter 7: Alzheimer's disease: A Biochemical Perspective	26
Chapter 8: The Role of Amyloid and Tau in Alzheimer's disease	29
Chapter 9: Vascular Dementia: The Impact of Blood Flow	32
Chapter 10: Frontotemporal Dementia: A Focus on Protein Aggregation	37
Chapter 11: Diet and Nutrition for Brain Health	42
Chapter 12: Exercise and Brain Health	47

Chapter 13: Sleep and Brain Health	51
Chapter 14: Genetics of Dementia: Risk Factors and Biomarkers	56
Chapter 15: The Impact of Lifestyle on Brain Health	60
Chapter 16: The Emotional Impact of Dementia	64
Chapter 17: Caring for Dementia Patients: A Biochemical Approach	68
Chapter 18: Effective Communication Techniques	72
Chapter 19: Daily Living and Care Strategies	76
Chapter 20: Early Signs and Symptoms of Dementia in Women	80
Chapter 21: Early Signs and Symptoms of Dementia in Men	83
Chapter 22: Tests for Diagnosing Dementia	86
Chapter 23: Managing Behavioral Changes	89
Chapter 24: Legal and Financial Considerations in Dementia Care	94
Chapter 25: Stages of Dementia, Life Expectancy, and Treatment	99
Chapter 26: Treatment for Lewy Body Dementia	103
Chapter 27: End-of-Life Care for Individuals with Dementia	107
Chapter 28: Seventy-seven (77) Facts about Dementia	111
Chapter 29: Future Trends in Dementia Care	121
Chapter 30: Personal Stories and Case Studies	126
Chapter 31: Hopes for the Future of Dementia Care	130
Chapter 32: Current Research and Future Directions in Treatment	136
Chapter 33: Conclusion and Call to Action	140
Glossary of Terms	145
Bibliography	153

INTRODUCTION

In recent years, dementia has emerged as a significant global health crisis, impacting millions of people and their families worldwide. As a biochemist, I have long been intrigued by the complex biological processes that underlie this devastating disease. Reclaiming Memories: A Guide to Preventing and Navigating Dementia aims to illuminate the biochemical mechanisms contributing to dementia while exploring potential strategies for prevention and treatment. This book is designed to provide researched insights that empower caregivers and enhance understanding among all readers.

The chapters within this book encompass a wide array of topics, ranging from the fundamental biochemistry of brain function to the latest research on emerging therapies. I have made a concerted effort to present complex scientific concepts in a clear and accessible manner, ensuring that this resource is suitable for both healthcare professionals and the general public.

A deeper understanding of the biochemistry of dementia is crucial for developing effective treatments. By investigating the underlying causes of this condition, we can identify new therapeutic targets and create more personalized approaches to care. This exploration not only advances our knowledge but also fosters hope for those affected by dementia.

Dementia encompasses various cognitive impairments that significantly affect memory, thinking, and daily functioning. As our population ages, the prevalence of dementia continues to rise, leading to profound emotional challenges—fear, confusion, sadness, and uncertainty about the future. Yet, amidst these challenges lies an opportunity for connection, understanding, and meaningful engagement.

Reclaiming Memories serves as a comprehensive resource for individuals living with dementia, their caregivers, and families. It is designed to empower readers with knowledge and practical strategies for navigating the complexities of dementia while fostering resilience and hope.

In addition to exploring the biochemical basis of dementia, this book covers:

- The various types of dementia and their symptoms, emphasizing the importance of early detection and understanding.
- The emotional impact of dementia on individuals and caregivers, along with strategies for managing these feelings.
- Effective communication techniques that enhance interactions and foster connections despite cognitive decline.
- Daily living strategies that promote independence and improve quality of life for individuals with dementia.
- Approaches for managing behavioral changes as the disease progresses.
- Legal and financial considerations essential for planning ahead and ensuring that individuals' wishes are respected.
- Future trends in dementia care, including advancements in research, community-based support models, and advocacy efforts.

Throughout this book, personal stories and case studies will illustrate the diverse experiences of those affected by dementia.

These narratives highlight the resilience of the human spirit and the profound connections that can emerge in the face of adversity.

Let us embark on this important conversation about dementia—one that honors the dignity of those affected while empowering individuals, families, and caregivers to embrace the journey ahead with hope and strength. Together, we can reclaim memories and foster a deeper understanding of brain health.

NB: Please refer to the glossary page of this book for seemingly complex or confusing terms.

Important Notice!
This book is intended for informational purposes only. For medical advice, diagnosis, or treatment, please consult your healthcare provider. While this book aims to empower you with knowledge to take proactive steps towards your health, it should not replace professional medical consultations.

ACKNOWLEDGMENTS

Writing Reclaiming Memories: A Guide to Preventing and Navigating Dementia has been a deeply rewarding journey, made possible by the support and contributions of many individuals and organizations. I would like to express my heartfelt gratitude to everyone who played a role in bringing this book to life.

First and foremost, I extend my sincere appreciation to the individuals living with dementia and their families who generously shared their stories and experiences with me. Your courage in facing this challenging journey has inspired me profoundly and shaped the content of this book. It is my hope that your voices resonate with others navigating similar paths.

I am immensely grateful to the healthcare professionals, researchers, and caregivers whose expertise and insights have enriched this work. Your dedication to improving the lives of those affected by dementia is commendable, and I appreciate the time you took to share your knowledge with me. Special thanks to Dr. Hope MacDaniels for his invaluable guidance and encouragement throughout this project.

To my family and friends, thank you for your unwavering support, patience, and understanding during the writing process. Your belief in my vision kept me motivated, even during the most challenging moments.

I would also like to acknowledge the organizations dedicated to dementia research and advocacy, such as the Alzheimer's Association and Alzheimer's Society. Your commitment to raising awareness and providing resources for individuals and families is vital in the fight against dementia.

Finally, I am grateful to my editor and publishing team for their expertise, encouragement, and dedication to bringing this book to fruition. Your insights have been instrumental in shaping this work into a resource that I hope will make a meaningful impact.

As we continue to navigate the complexities of dementia care together, let us remember that our collective efforts can foster understanding, compassion, and hope for those affected by this condition. Thank you all for being part of this journey.

CHAPTER 1: UNDERSTANDING DEMENTIA: A BIOCHEMICAL PERSPECTIVE

Dementia is a complex syndrome characterized by a progressive decline in cognitive function, significantly impacting memory, reasoning, and daily living activities. In this book, the biochemical mechanisms underlying dementia will be examined while providing insights into its pathophysiology and potential interventions.

Essentially, dementia is not a single disease but rather a general term that describes a group of symptoms affecting memory, thinking, and social abilities severe enough to interfere with everyday life. It is important to note that dementia is not a normal part of aging; while the risk increases with age, many older adults live without any signs of cognitive decline (National Institute on Aging).

Defining Dementia

Dementia encompasses various neurodegenerative disorders, with Alzheimer's disease (AD) being the most common of cases. It is a composite and multifaceted condition that affects millions of individuals worldwide, profoundly impacting their cognitive abilities and daily functioning. It is essential to understand what dementia is, it's various types, symptoms, and progression to navigate the challenges it presents effectively.

According to statistical data from Alzheimer's Disease International, there is a steady increment in cases of dementia yearly in low and middle income countries compared to high income countries:

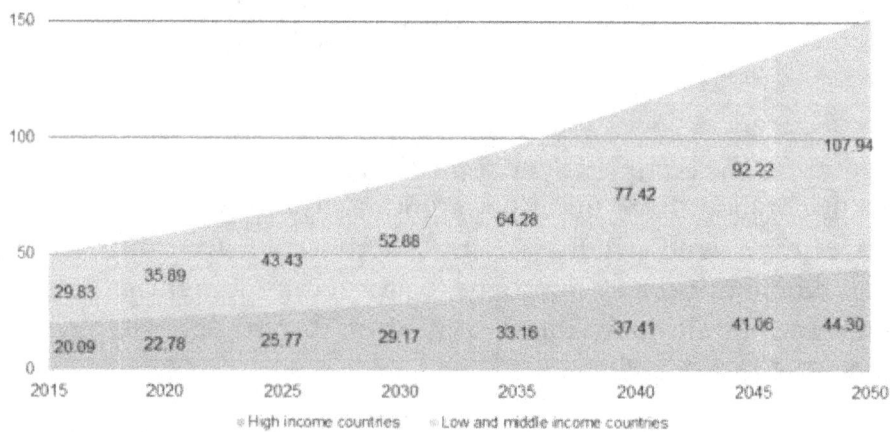

Types of Dementia

There are several types of dementia, each with distinct characteristics and underlying causes:

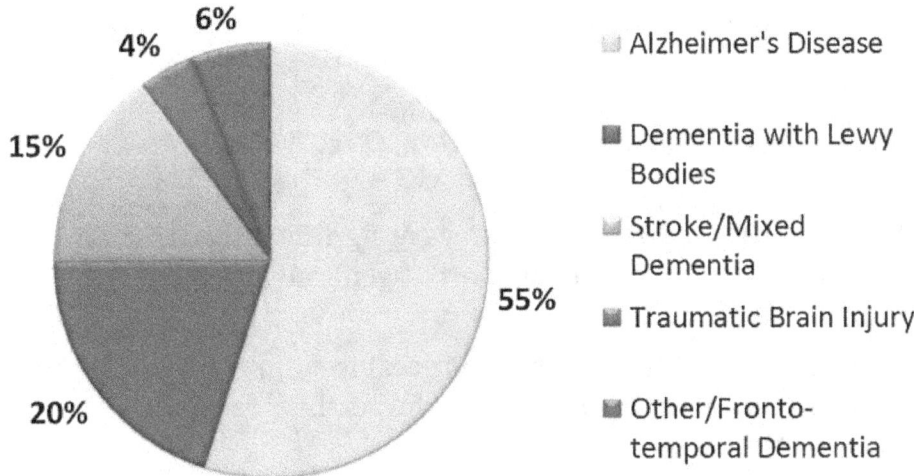

1. Alzheimer's Disease: The most common form of dementia, accounting for approximately 60-80% of cases. It typically begins with memory loss and progresses to difficulties in reasoning and language.

2. Vascular Dementia: This type results from reduced blood flow to the brain, often following strokes. Symptoms can vary widely depending on the areas affected.

3. Lewy Body Dementia: Characterized by fluctuations in alertness, visual hallucinations, and motor symptoms similar to Parkinson's disease. This type can present unique challenges due to its combination of cognitive and physical symptoms.

4. Frontotemporal Dementia: Involves degeneration of the frontal and temporal lobes of the brain, leading to changes in personality and behavior as well as difficulties with language.

5. Mixed Dementia: A condition where an individual exhibits characteristics of more than one type of dementia, commonly Alzheimer's disease combined with vascular dementia.

Symptoms and Stages

The symptoms of dementia can vary significantly depending on the type and stage of the disease but generally include:

- Memory Loss: Often the first noticeable symptom, particularly short-term memory loss (e.g., forgetting recent events or conversations).
- Communication Difficulties: Struggles with finding words or following conversations.
- Disorientation: Confusion about time or place, often leading to feelings of being lost even in familiar environments.
- Behavioral Changes: Mood swings, anxiety, agitation, or inappropriate behavior may emerge as the condition progresses (Alzheimer's Society).
- Difficulty with Daily Tasks: Challenges in planning or completing familiar tasks like cooking or managing finances.

Stages of Dementia

Dementia typically progresses through three stages:

1. Early Stage (Mild): Individuals may still maintain independence but begin experiencing forgetfulness and minor confusion. It is often during this stage that families notice changes and may seek help.

2. Middle Stage (Moderate): Symptoms become more pronounced; individuals may require assistance with daily activities as memory loss and confusion increase. Behavioral

changes are also common at this stage (Alzheimer's Society).

3. Late Stage (Severe): Individuals may lose the ability to communicate effectively and require full-time care. They may not recognize loved ones and experience significant physical challenges.

These symptoms and stages will be further discussed in subsequent chapters. These symptomatic progression typically follows stages from mild cognitive impairment (MCI) to severe dementia, where individuals may lose basic functional abilities. Early diagnosis is important for effective management.

The Biochemical Basis of Dementia

Neurodegeneration

Neurodegeneration is central to dementia's pathology. The implicated primary biochemical factors include:

- **Protein Misfolding**: In Alzheimer's disease (AD), amyloid-beta (Aβ) proteins aggregate to form plaques that disrupt neuronal function. Tau proteins become hyperphosphorylated, leading to neurofibrillary tangles that impair microtubule stability and transport within neurons.

- **Oxidative Stress:** This imbalance between free radicals and antioxidants leads to cellular damage. Oxidative stress is implicated in the early stages of AD and contributes to neuronal death.

- **Inflammation:** Neuroinflammation plays a significant role in AD progression. Activated microglia release cytokines that can exacerbate neuronal damage.

Neurotransmitter Imbalances

Neurotransmitters are essential for neuronal communication. In dementia, imbalances can lead to cognitive decline (where there is 'misunderstanding' or no communication at all among the neurons):

- Acetylcholine: Deficits in this neurotransmitter are particularly notable in AD, where cholinergic dysfunction is prevalent.

- Glutamate: While essential for learning and memory, excessive glutamate can lead to excitotoxicity—damaging neurons through overstimulation.

Summary

This introductory chapter ushers us in into the complexities of dementia. Elements and terms mentioned will be discussed more as we progress into subsequent chapters.

A good understanding of dementia from a biochemical perspective illuminates its complexities. As we continue our journey through this book, we will probe deeper into amyloid and tau proteins' roles in Alzheimer's disease, investigate genetic risk factors for dementia, and discuss lifestyle choices that can impact brain health. Together, these insights will contribute to a holistic understanding of dementia from a biochemist's perspective.

"The pathogenesis of Alzheimer's disease involves a multifactorial interplay of genetic, biochemical, and environmental factors" (Griciuc & Tanzi, 2021).

CHAPTER 2: RISK FACTORS AND PREVENTION STRATEGIES

A good understanding of the risk factors associated with dementia is imperative for developing effective prevention strategies. As the prevalence of dementia continues to rise globally, identifying lifestyle and biological factors that can influence its onset becomes increasingly important. This chapter explores key risk factors for dementia and outlines actionable strategies that individuals can adopt to potentially reduce their risk.

Fundamental Risk Factors for Dementia

Research has identified several modifiable and non-modifiable risk factors that contribute to the development of dementia:

1. **Age:** Age is the most significant non-modifiable risk factor for dementia. The likelihood of developing dementia increases significantly after the age of 65, with risk doubling every five years thereafter (Alzheimer's Association, 2021).

2. **Genetics:** Family history plays a role in the risk of developing certain types of dementia, particularly Alzheimer's disease. Genetic factors can influence susceptibility, although they are not deterministic (National Institute on Aging).

3. **Vascular Risk Factors**: Conditions such as hypertension, diabetes, dyslipidemia, and obesity are consistently linked to an increased risk of dementia. These conditions can lead to vascular damage in the brain, contributing to cognitive decline (Yaffe et al., 2008).

4. **Depression**: Individuals with a history of depression are at a higher risk for cognitive impairment and dementia. Depression may contribute to neurodegenerative processes or serve as an early indicator of cognitive decline (Kessing et al., 2010).

5. **Social Isolation**: Loneliness and social isolation have been associated with an increased risk of dementia. Engaging in social activities can provide cognitive stimulation and emotional support, both vital for brain health (Holt-Lunstad et al., 2010).

Promising Prevention Strategies

While some risk factors cannot be changed, research suggests that lifestyle modifications can significantly reduce the risk of developing dementia. The following are some evidence-based strategies:

1. **Cognitive Activity**: Engaging in mentally stimulating activities—such as reading, puzzles, or learning new skills—can enhance cognitive reserve and potentially delay the onset of dementia. Studies show that individuals who participate in

cognitive activities throughout their lives exhibit lower rates of cognitive decline compared to those who do not (Valenzuela & Sachdev, 2006).

2. **Physical Activity**: Regular physical exercise is associated with a lower risk of cognitive decline and dementia. Exercise improves cardiovascular health, which is crucial for maintaining optimal brain function. The Lancet Commission on Dementia Prevention notes that sustained physical activity in midlife can protect against dementia by reducing obesity and cardiovascular risks (Livingston et al., 2020).

3. **Healthy Diet**: A diet rich in antioxidants, polyunsaturated fats, and whole foods—such as the Mediterranean diet—has been linked to better cognitive health. This diet emphasizes fruits, vegetables, whole grains, fish, and healthy fats while limiting processed foods and sugars (Scarmeas et al., 2006).

4. **Social Engagement**: Maintaining strong social connections is vital for cognitive health. Participating in community activities or support groups can reduce feelings of isolation and promote mental well-being (Cattan et al., 2005).

5. **Managing Vascular Health**: Controlling vascular risk factors through regular check-ups and lifestyle changes—such as maintaining healthy blood pressure and cholesterol levels—can significantly reduce the risk of developing dementia (Yaffe et al., 2008).

6. **Addressing Hearing Loss**: Recent studies suggest that untreated hearing loss may increase the risk of cognitive decline. Using hearing aids or other assistive devices can help mitigate this risk by improving communication and social interaction (Lin et al., 2011).

Summary

The potential to prevent or delay the onset of dementia through lifestyle modifications is promising. Through the understanding of the key risk factors associated with dementia and implementing strategies such as engaging in cognitive activities, maintaining physical fitness, following a healthy diet, fostering social connections, managing vascular health, and addressing hearing loss, individuals can take proactive steps toward safeguarding their cognitive health.

Through the prioritization of these prevention strategies, we can foster healthier aging and improve overall quality of life while navigating the complexities associated with dementia care.

CHAPTER 3: THE BRAIN: A MARVEL OF BIOCHEMISTRY

The human brain, a complex organ weighing approximately three pounds, is the command center of our bodies. It is responsible for everything from our thoughts and emotions to our movements and senses. At its core, the brain is a marvel of biochemistry, a network of cells and molecules that work together to create the intricate tapestry of our consciousness.

The Brain's Structure and Functions

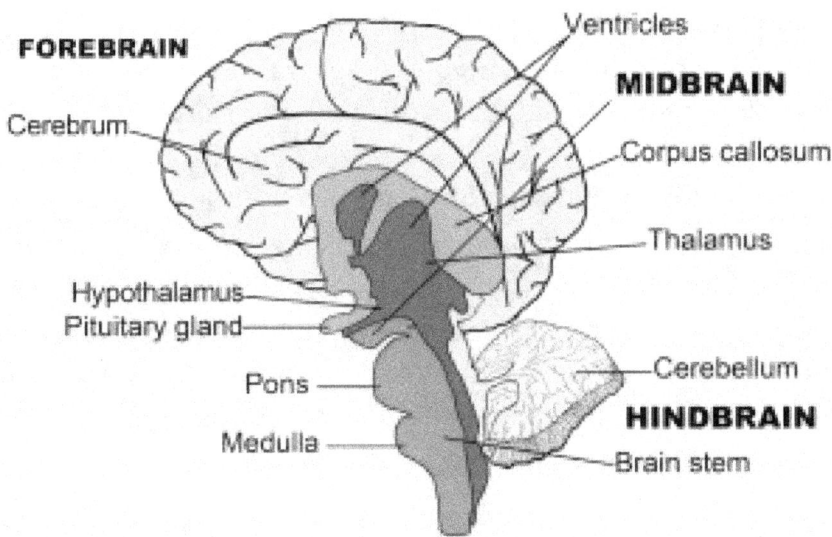

The human brain, weighing approximately three pounds, is a complex organ composed primarily of neural tissue. It is divided into three main structures: the cerebrum, cerebellum, and brainstem. Each of these components plays a crucial role in various bodily functions, including movement, cognition, and emotional regulation. The cerebrum, the largest part of the brain, is responsible for higher cognitive functions such as thinking, problem-solving, and controlling voluntary movements. It is further divided into four lobes: frontal, temporal, parietal, and occipital, each with distinct functions related to personality, sensory processing, and motor control.

The brain communicates with the body through a network of billions of neurons that transmit electrical and chemical signals. This sophisticated communication system allows the brain to process sensory information, regulate bodily functions, and coordinate responses to environmental stimuli. The brainstem connects the brain to the spinal cord and controls vital life functions such as breathing and heart rate.

The Biochemical Basis of Brain Function

Maintaining brain health involves several key biochemical processes that are essential for its optimal functioning:

1. **Neurotransmitter Regulation:**

Neurotransmitters are chemical messengers that facilitate communication between neurons. Key neurotransmitters include dopamine, serotonin, and norepinephrine. For example, dopamine plays a critical role in motivation and reward pathways; its dysregulation is linked to conditions such as Parkinson's disease and addiction.

2. **Neuroplasticity:**

Neuroplasticity refers to the brain's ability to reorganize itself by forming new neural connections throughout life. This process is vital for learning and memory. Research indicates that engaging in mentally stimulating activities can enhance neuroplasticity and improve cognitive function.

3. Energy Metabolism:

The brain requires a significant amount of energy to function properly, utilizing glucose as its primary energy source. Mitochondria within neurons convert glucose into adenosine triphosphate (ATP), which powers cellular processes. Disruptions in energy metabolism can lead to neurodegenerative diseases.

4. Oxidative Stress Response:

The brain is particularly vulnerable to oxidative stress due to its high oxygen consumption. Antioxidants play a crucial role in neutralizing free radicals that can damage cells. A diet rich in antioxidants (e.g., vitamins C and E) has been associated with better cognitive health.

5. Inflammation Regulation:

Chronic inflammation in the brain can contribute to neurodegenerative diseases like Alzheimer's disease. The presence of inflammatory cytokines can affect neuronal function and survival. Research suggests that anti-inflammatory agents may help mitigate these effects.

Summary

The brain is a complex and fascinating organ that is the product of billions of years of evolution. Its biochemical processes are essential for our thoughts, emotions, and behaviors. Through our understanding of the biochemistry of the brain, we can gain a deeper appreciation for the incredible complexity of human consciousness.

CHAPTER 4: NEUROTRANSMITTERS: THE BRAIN'S CHEMICAL MESSENGERS

Neurotransmitters are the chemical messengers that allow neurons to communicate with each other. These molecules are stored in tiny vesicles within the neuron and are released into the synaptic cleft, the space between two neurons, when a neuron fires. Neurotransmitters bind to receptors on the surface of the receiving neuron, triggering a variety of responses.

Types of Neurotransmitters

There are many different types of neurotransmitters, each with its own unique functions. Some of the most important neurotransmitters include:

- **Dopamine:** Dopamine is involved in reward, pleasure, and motivation. It is also important for movement and learning.
- **Serotonin:** Serotonin is involved in mood, appetite, and sleep. It is also important for cognitive function.

- **Norepinephrine:** Norepinephrine is involved in the fight-or-flight response. It is also important for attention and arousal.
- **Glutamate:** Glutamate is the most abundant excitatory neurotransmitter in the brain. It is involved in learning and memory.
- **GABA:** GABA is the most abundant inhibitory neurotransmitter in the brain. It is involved in relaxation and sleep.

Central Role of Glutamate Metabolism in the Maintenance of Nitrogen Homeostasis in Normal and Hyperammonemic Brain

The central role of glutamate metabolism is crucial for maintaining nitrogen homeostasis in both normal and hyperammonemic brains, as glutamate serves as a key amino acid involved in various metabolic pathways. In the brain, glutamate exists at high concentrations, primarily functioning as an excitatory neurotransmitter while also participating in nitrogen metabolism through its conversion to glutamine via glutamine synthetase, which helps regulate ammonia levels and prevent neurotoxicity. Under hyperammonemic conditions, such as those seen in liver dysfunction, the metabolism of glutamate shifts towards increased synthesis of glutamine, effectively buffering excess ammonia and facilitating the production of 5-carbon units through the stimulation of anaplerotic enzymes like pyruvate carboxylase. This dynamic interplay between glutamate and glutamine underscores the importance of glutamate not only in neurotransmitter cycling but also in nitrogen balance, highlighting its protective role against the detrimental effects of elevated ammonia levels on brain function:

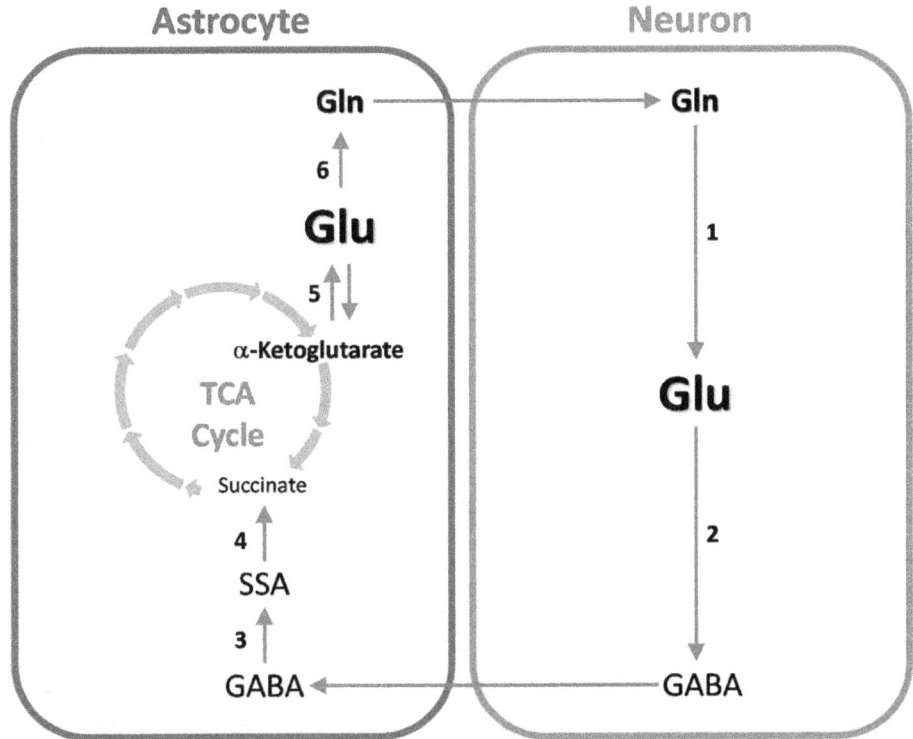

Neurotransmitter Imbalances and Brain Health

Imbalances in neurotransmitter levels can lead to a variety of neurological and psychiatric disorders. For example, low levels of dopamine are associated with Parkinson's disease, while low levels of serotonin are associated with depression. High levels of glutamate can lead to excitotoxicity, a process that can damage neurons.

Summary

Neurotransmitters are essential for brain function. They allow neurons to communicate with each other, enabling us to think, feel, and act. Imbalances in neurotransmitter levels can lead to a variety of neurological and psychiatric disorders. Understanding the role of neurotransmitters in brain health is important for developing new treatments for these disorders.

CHAPTER 5: NEUROTRANSMITTERS AND COGNITIVE DECLINE

As mentioned in the previous chapter, neurotransmitters play a pivotal role in cognitive functions, and their dysregulation is a hallmark of Alzheimer's disease (AD). This chapter probes deeper into the major neurotransmitter systems involved in AD—primarily acetylcholine, glutamate, dopamine, and norepinephrine—and their contributions to cognitive decline.

The Cholinergic System

The cholinergic hypothesis posits that a deficit in acetylcholine (ACh) is central to the cognitive impairment seen in AD. ACh is crucial for learning and memory, and its levels are significantly reduced in AD patients due to the degeneration of cholinergic neurons in the basal forebrain. Research indicates that "the loss and dysfunction of cholinergic neurons are among the initial signs of AD pathogenesis" (Petersen et al., 2011).

Cholinesterase inhibitors, which increase ACh availability at synapses, have been shown to improve cognitive function in

AD patients. As noted by Cummings et al. (2022), "these drugs validate the cholinergic system as an important therapeutic target" for AD treatment.

The Glutamatergic System

Glutamate, the primary excitatory neurotransmitter in the brain, is also implicated in AD pathology. The glutamatergic hypothesis links cognitive decline to neuronal damage caused by overactivation of N-methyl-D-aspartate (NMDA) receptors. Sustained low-level activation of these receptors can lead to excitotoxicity, contributing to neuronal death.

Research has shown that "excessive release of glutamate into the synaptic cleft contributes to cell death and neuronal damage" when Aβ plaques are present (Hasselmo & Sarter, 2011). This suggests that restoring glutamate balance may be crucial for mitigating cognitive decline:

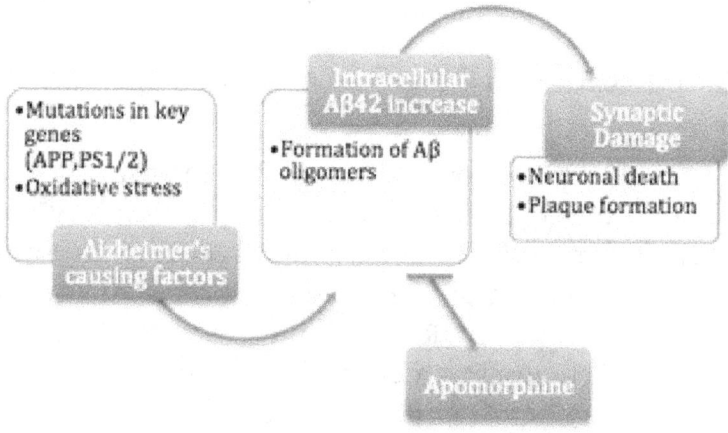

Dopamine and Norepinephrine

Dopamine and norepinephrine are also critical for cognitive function but are often overlooked in discussions about AD. The degeneration of dopaminergic neurons in the ventral tegmental area (VTA) has been linked to memory deficits in AD patients. According to recent findings, "the degeneration of dopaminergic neurons causes significant memory impairments" (Xiong et al., 2004).

Norepinephrine, produced by neurons in the locus coeruleus, plays a role in attention and arousal. Recent studies indicate that alterations in noradrenergic signaling may contribute to cognitive decline associated with aging and AD. Mather et al. (2023) emphasize that "changes in brain regions producing norepinephrine are linked to episodic memory," highlighting its importance for long-term memory retention.

The Interplay between Neurotransmitters

The interplay between these neurotransmitter systems is complex. For instance, cholinergic deficits can lead to increased glutamatergic activity, exacerbating excitotoxicity. As noted by Vermeiren et al. (2023), "combined alterations in brain neurotransmitter systems occur across various dementia subtypes," indicating a shared biochemical landscape that complicates treatment approaches.

Moreover, research has shown that deficiencies in neurotransmitter precursors can further impair cognitive function. For example, low levels of amino acid precursors necessary for neurotransmitter synthesis have been observed in both AD and mild cognitive impairment (MCI) patients.

Summary

Neurotransmitter dysregulation is a fundamental aspect of Alzheimer's disease that contributes significantly to cognitive decline. Understanding these systems' roles provides critical insights into potential therapeutic strategies aimed at restoring neurotransmitter balance. In subsequent chapters, we will explore genetic risk factors associated with dementia and lifestyle choices that can influence brain health.

> "The interplay between various neurotransmitter systems underscores the complexity of cognitive decline in Alzheimer's disease" (Cummings et al., 2022).

CHAPTER 6: ENERGY METABOLISM IN THE BRAIN

As mentioned in earlier chapter of this book, the brain is a highly active organ that requires a constant supply of energy to function properly. This energy is derived primarily from the metabolism of glucose, a simple sugar. Glucose is transported into brain cells and broken down through a series of biochemical reactions known as glycolysis, the Krebs cycle, and oxidative phosphorylation.

Glucose Metabolism

Glucose is the primary fuel source for the brain. It is transported into brain cells through a special transporter protein called the glucose transporter 1 (GLUT1). Once inside the cell, glucose is broken down through glycolysis, a process that yields pyruvate. Pyruvate can then enter the mitochondria, where it is further metabolized through the Krebs cycle and oxidative phosphorylation:

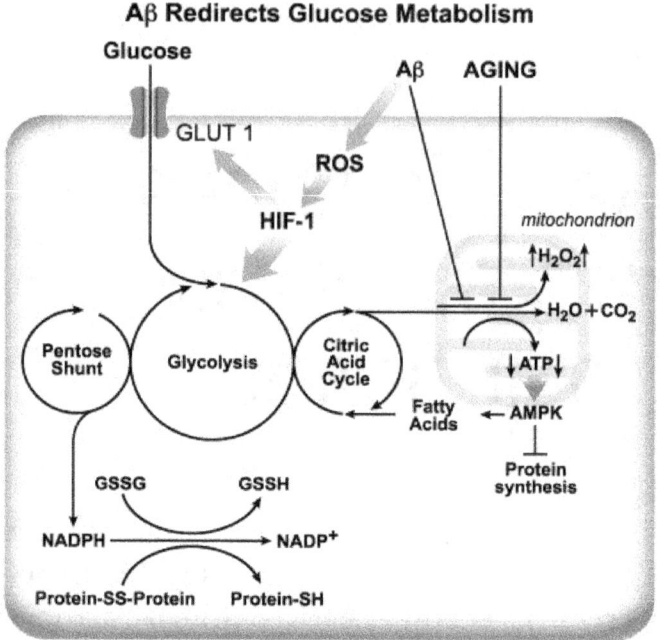

Mitochondrial Dysfunction and Brain Health

Mitochondria are the "powerhouses" of the cell. They are responsible for producing energy in the form of adenosine triphosphate (ATP). Mitochondrial dysfunction, or the inability of mitochondria to produce sufficient ATP, has been implicated in a number of neurodegenerative diseases, including Alzheimer's disease and Parkinson's disease.

Summary

Energy metabolism is essential for brain function. Glucose is the primary fuel source for the brain, and it is broken down through a series of biochemical reactions to produce energy. Mitochondrial dysfunction can lead to neurodegenerative diseases. Understanding the role of energy metabolism in brain health is important for developing new treatments for these disorders.

CHAPTER 7: ALZHEIMER'S DISEASE: A BIOCHEMICAL PERSPECTIVE

As earlier mentioned, Alzheimer's disease (AD) is a progressive neurodegenerative disorder characterized by memory loss, cognitive decline, and behavioral changes. It is the most common cause of dementia, affecting millions of people worldwide.

Alzheimer's Disease

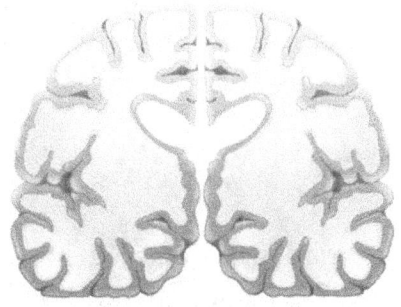
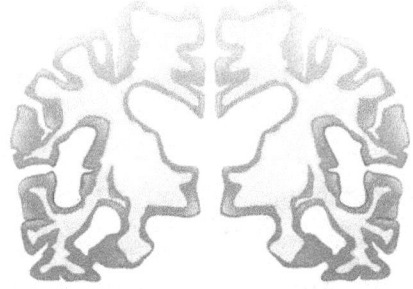

Healthy Brain   Alzheimer's Disease

The Biochemistry of Alzheimer's disease

At the biochemical level, Alzheimer's disease (AD) is characterized by the formation of amyloid plaques and neurofibrillary tangles. Amyloid plaques are composed of beta-amyloid protein, a fragment of a larger protein called amyloid precursor protein (APP). Neurofibrillary tangles are composed of hyperphosphorylated tau protein, a protein that is normally involved in stabilizing microtubules.

The exact cause of AD is unknown, but it is believed to be a complex interplay of genetic, environmental, and lifestyle factors. Several hypotheses have been proposed, including:

- **Amyloid Cascade Hypothesis:** This hypothesis suggests that the accumulation of beta-amyloid protein in the brain is the primary cause of AD.
- **Tau Hypothesis:** This hypothesis suggests that the accumulation of tau protein in the brain is the primary cause of AD.

- **Inflammation Hypothesis:** This hypothesis suggests that chronic inflammation in the brain plays a role in the development of AD.
- **Oxidative Stress Hypothesis:** This hypothesis suggests that oxidative stress, or damage to cells caused by reactive oxygen species, plays a role in the development of AD.

Summary

Alzheimer's disease is a complex neurodegenerative disorder characterized by the formation of amyloid plaques and neurofibrillary tangles. The exact cause of AD is unknown, but it is believed to be a complex interplay of genetic, environmental, and lifestyle factors. Understanding the biochemistry of AD is important for developing new treatments for this devastating disease.

CHAPTER 8: THE ROLE OF AMYLOID AND TAU IN ALZHEIMER'S DISEASE

Alzheimer's disease (AD) is characterized by the accumulation of two hallmark proteins: amyloid-beta (Aβ) and tau. Understanding the interplay between these proteins is essential for unraveling the pathogenesis of AD. This chapter, a sequel to the previous one explores the biochemical roles of Aβ and tau, their interactions, and their contributions to neurodegeneration.

Amyloid-Beta: The Trigger

Aβ is a peptide derived from the amyloid precursor protein (APP) and is primarily associated with the formation of extracellular plaques in the brains of AD patients. The amyloid cascade hypothesis posits that Aβ accumulation is the initial event leading to neuronal damage and cognitive decline. According to Bloom (2014), "Aβ is upstream of tau in AD pathogenesis and triggers the conversion of tau from a normal to a toxic state".

Research has shown that soluble forms of Aβ can induce

synaptic dysfunction and neuron death, which are critical for memory impairment in AD. This suggests that Aβ not only accumulates but also actively participates in disease progression by promoting tau toxicity.

Tau: The Bullet

Tau is a microtubule-associated protein that stabilizes neuronal axons under normal conditions. In AD, tau becomes hyperphosphorylated, leading to the formation of neurofibrillary tangles (NFTs) within neurons. These tangles disrupt microtubule stability, impairing axonal transport and ultimately resulting in cell death.

The relationship between Aβ and tau is complex; while Aβ initiates tau pathology, tau itself exacerbates Aβ toxicity. As noted by Busche and Hyman (2020), "Both pathologies have synergistic effects," suggesting that targeting either protein alone may not be sufficient for effective treatment.

The Interplay between Amyloid and Tau

Recent studies indicate that Aβ and tau may begin as independent processes in spatially disconnected brain regions. For instance, amyloid accumulation typically starts in the neocortex, while tau pathology often begins in the medial temporal lobe. This spatial discordance complicates our understanding of their interactions.

However, evidence suggests that local interactions between Aβ and tau can lead to widespread tau propagation throughout the brain. In some cases, individuals with a genetic predisposition (such as APOE ε4 carriers) exhibit a "tau-first" pathology, where tau accumulation precedes significant Aβ deposition.

This highlights the need for personalized approaches in understanding AD progression.

Implications for Treatment

The complex relationship between Aβ and tau has profound implications for therapeutic strategies. While many clinical trials have focused on targeting Aβ alone, the synergy between these two proteins suggests that combined approaches may yield better outcomes. As noted by researchers, "successful therapeutic intervention for AD would benefit from detecting these species before plaques, tangles, and cognitive impairment become evident".

Summary

Understanding the roles of amyloid-beta and tau in Alzheimer's disease is essential for developing effective therapies. Their interplay not only drives neurodegeneration but also complicates treatment strategies. As we move forward in this book, we will explore genetic risk factors associated with dementia and how lifestyle choices can influence brain health.

"The defining features of Alzheimer disease include conspicuous changes in both brain histology and behavior" (Bloom, 2014).

CHAPTER 9: VASCULAR DEMENTIA: THE IMPACT OF BLOOD FLOW

Vascular dementia is a significant form of cognitive decline that arises from impaired blood flow to the brain, leading to brain cell damage and eventual cognitive impairment. It is the second most common type of dementia after Alzheimer's disease, and its prevalence is expected to rise as the population ages. Understanding the mechanisms behind vascular dementia, particularly the role of blood flow, is crucial for prevention and management.

Causes and Mechanisms

The primary cause of vascular dementia is reduced blood flow to brain tissue, which can occur due to various conditions. These include:

Stroke: A sudden blockage or rupture of blood vessels can lead to immediate cognitive decline. According to the National Institute on Aging, "major strokes can also increase the risk for dementia, but not everyone who has had a stroke will develop dementia".

Chronic conditions: Conditions such as high blood pressure, diabetes, and high cholesterol can damage blood vessels over time, leading to a gradual decline in blood supply to the brain. The Mayo Clinic notes that "vascular dementia results from conditions that damage blood vessels and block blood flow to your brain".

Mini-strokes: Also known as transient ischemic attacks (TIAs), these small strokes can cause cumulative damage that contributes to vascular dementia. The NHS emphasizes that "lots of mini-strokes... cause tiny but widespread damage to the brain".

Dr. Juebin Huang from the University of Mississippi Medical Center explains that "the cause is usually strokes, either a few large ones or many small ones," highlighting the importance of both acute and chronic vascular events in the development of this condition.

Symptoms and Diagnosis

Symptoms of vascular dementia can vary widely depending on which areas of the brain are affected. Common symptoms include:

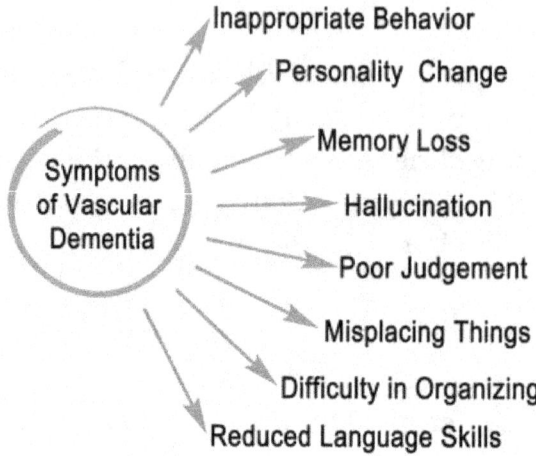

- Confusion and difficulty concentrating
- Slowed thinking and problems with organization
- Memory loss that may be less pronounced than in Alzheimer's disease
- Physical symptoms such as weakness or tremors

The onset of symptoms may be sudden following a stroke or gradual due to cumulative vascular damage. According to Johns Hopkins Medicine, "the effect of decreased or no blood flow on the brain depends on the size and location of the area affected". This variability makes diagnosis challenging, as symptoms often overlap with other forms of dementia.

Risk Factors

Several risk factors contribute to the likelihood of developing vascular dementia. These include:

- **Age**: The risk increases significantly for individuals over 65.

- **Lifestyle factors**: Smoking, poor diet, lack of exercise, and excessive alcohol consumption can all elevate risk.
- **Medical conditions**: Hypertension, diabetes, and heart disease are significant contributors.

The NHS warns that "controlling these factors may help lower your chances of developing vascular dementia". Dr. Huang also notes that eliminating stroke risk factors may delay or prevent further damage associated with vascular dementia.

Treatment and Management

Currently, there is no cure for vascular dementia; however, treatment focuses on managing symptoms and underlying conditions. Lifestyle changes play a crucial role in slowing disease progression. The Cleveland Clinic suggests that managing conditions like heart disease and diabetes is essential for preventing further cognitive decline.

Medications may be prescribed to address specific symptoms or underlying health issues. For instance, anticoagulants may be used to prevent further strokes in at-risk patients. Additionally, surgical interventions aimed at improving blood flow may be considered in certain cases.

Summary

Vascular dementia represents a complex interplay between reduced blood flow and cognitive decline. Understanding its causes—primarily related to vascular health—can inform prevention strategies and management approaches. As research continues to evolve, it remains critical for individuals at risk to adopt healthier lifestyles and seek regular medical advice to mitigate their chances of developing this debilitating condition.

CHAPTER 10: FRONTOTEMPORAL DEMENTIA: A FOCUS ON PROTEIN AGGREGATION

Frontotemporal dementia (FTD) is a complex neurodegenerative disorder characterized by progressive degeneration of the frontal and temporal lobes of the brain. This condition often manifests in individuals *between the ages of 45 and 65*, leading to significant changes in personality, behavior, and language capabilities. Recent discoveries in the field of protein aggregation have shed light on the underlying mechanisms of FTD and opened new avenues for diagnosis and treatment.

Frontotemporal Dementia

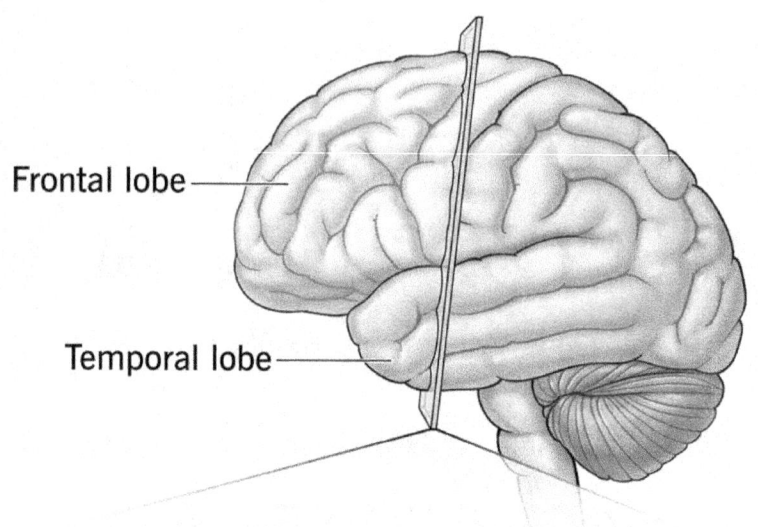

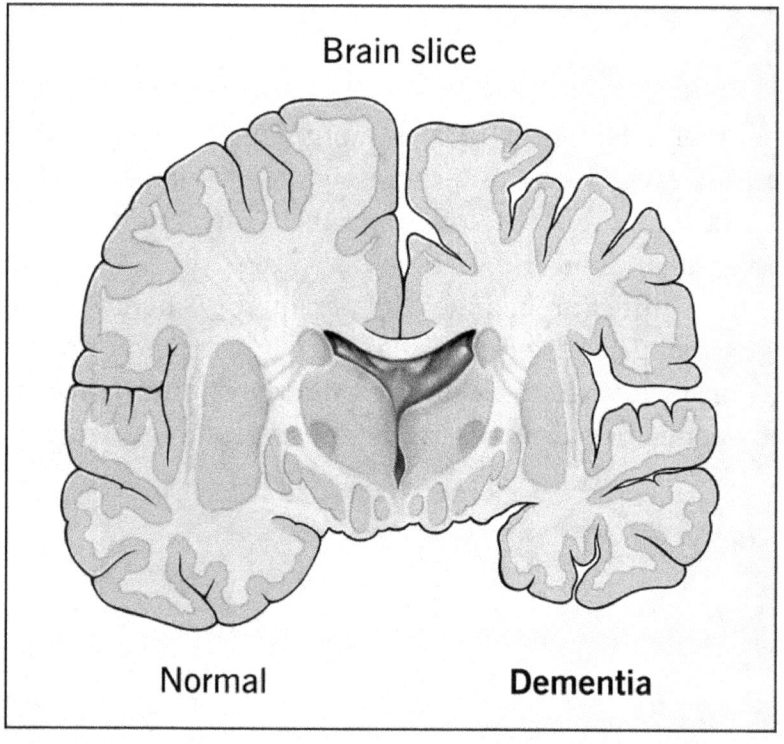

Understanding Protein Aggregation in FTD

Protein aggregation is a hallmark of many neurodegenerative diseases, including FTD. In these disorders, proteins misfold and accumulate into structures known as amyloids, which disrupt normal cellular functions. Traditionally, proteins such as tau and TDP-43 have been implicated in FTD; however, recent research has identified a novel protein, TAF15, as a significant contributor to the pathology of this disease.

In a groundbreaking study published in Nature, researchers from the Medical Research Council (MRC) Laboratory of Molecular Biology utilized cryo-electron microscopy (cryo-EM) to analyze brain samples from individuals with early-onset dementia. They discovered that TAF15 forms aggregated structures in cases previously thought to be associated primarily with the protein FUS. Research lead Benjamin Ryskeldi-Falcon stated, "This discovery transforms our understanding of the molecular basis of frontotemporal dementia". The identification of TAF15 not only challenges existing assumptions but also provides a new target for diagnostic and therapeutic strategies.

The Role of Neuroinflammation

Neuroinflammation is another critical aspect associated with FTD. Studies have shown that neuroinflammation co-localizes with protein aggregation across various forms of frontotemporal dementia. Bevan-Jones et al. demonstrated through positron emission tomography (PET) that activated microglia—immune cells in the brain—are significantly involved in the inflammatory response observed in FTD patients. This relationship suggests that both protein aggregation and inflammation may interact to exacerbate the clinical manifestations of dementia.

Dr. James Giordano from Georgetown University commented on the implications of these findings, noting that "this study further examined the possibility that additional abnormal proteins may be contributory to the neuropathological process of frontotemporal lobar degeneration". This highlights the need for a multifaceted approach when considering treatment options for FTD.

Implications for Diagnosis and Treatment

The discovery of TAF15 aggregates opens new pathways for developing diagnostic tools and targeted therapies. With advanced imaging techniques like cryo-EM, researchers can now screen for abnormal protein aggregates in larger populations, potentially leading to earlier detection and intervention strategies. Bernardino Ghetti, a lead neuropathologist involved in the study, emphasized that this breakthrough "recognizes TAF15 as a potential target for the development of diagnostic and therapeutic strategies".

Moreover, understanding how TAF15 aggregates relate to other neurodegenerative diseases such as amyotrophic lateral sclerosis (ALS) may provide insights into overlapping pathologies. The presence of identical TAF15 aggregates in individuals exhibiting both FTD and motor neuron disease raises intriguing questions about shared mechanisms between these disorders.

Summary

The recent advancements in understanding protein aggregation in frontotemporal dementia underscore the complexity of this disease and its interaction with neuroinflammation. Identifying TAF15 as a key player not only enhances our understanding of FTD's molecular underpinnings but also paves the way for innovative diagnostic and therapeutic approaches. As research continues to evolve, it is crucial to explore these findings further to improve outcomes for individuals affected by this debilitating condition.

CHAPTER 11: DIET AND NUTRITION FOR BRAIN HEALTH

The relationship between diet and brain health has garnered significant attention in recent years, with extensive research indicating that our food choices can profoundly impact cognitive function and mental well-being. This chapter explores the key dietary patterns and nutrients linked to optimal brain health, supported by recent studies and expert insights.

The Role of a Ketogenic Diet in the Treatment of Dementia in Type 2 Diabetes Mellitus Patients

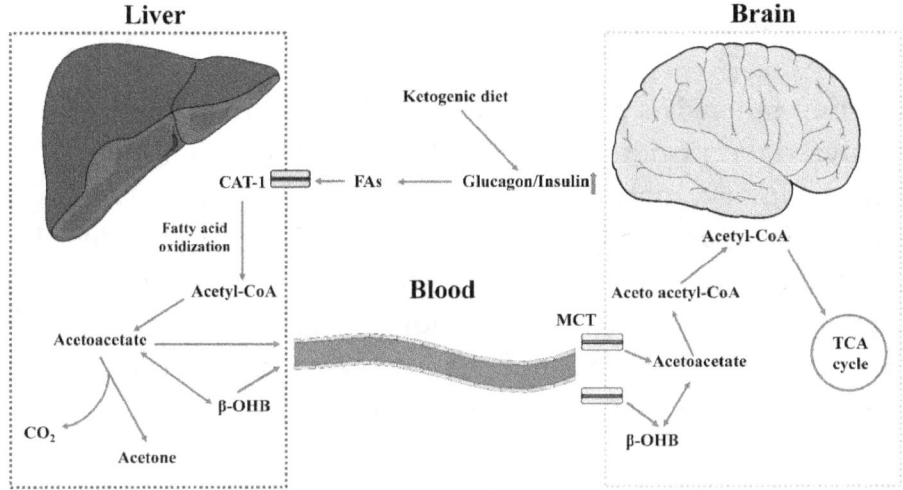

The ketogenic diet (KD), characterized by high fat and low carbohydrate intake, has emerged as a promising dietary intervention for individuals with Type 2 Diabetes Mellitus (T2DM) experiencing cognitive decline or dementia. Research indicates that T2DM shares common pathological mechanisms with dementia, particularly involving impaired insulin signaling and altered glucose metabolism in the brain, which can lead to neuroinflammation and cognitive deficits. The KD induces a metabolic state known as ketosis, where the body utilizes ketone bodies as an alternative energy source, potentially enhancing neuronal function and protecting against oxidative stress. A review highlights that ketone bodies may improve synaptic plasticity and reduce neuroinflammation, thereby offering neuroprotective effects that could mitigate the progression of dementia in T2DM patients. As noted in recent studies, implementing the KD may provide a viable strategy for managing cognitive decline associated with diabetes, emphasizing the need for further research to establish clear dietary guidelines for this population.

The Importance of a Balanced Diet

A comprehensive study published in Nature Mental Health analyzed data from nearly 182,000 participants and identified four primary dietary patterns: *starch-free*, *vegetarian*, *high-protein low-fiber*, and *balanced diets*. The findings revealed that individuals adhering to a balanced diet—characterized by a variety of fruits, vegetables, whole grains, lean proteins, and healthy fats—exhibited superior cognitive functions and mental health compared to those following other dietary patterns.

Researchers noted that the balanced diet group not only had higher levels of gray matter in crucial brain regions but also reported better mental health outcomes. This suggests that a diverse intake of nutrients plays a vital role in maintaining cognitive health. "A healthy, balanced diet was linked to superior brain health," stated the research team from the University of Warwick, highlighting the profound connection between dietary choices and cognitive function.

Key Dietary Patterns for Brain Health

Several eating patterns have been specifically associated with improved brain health:

- Mediterranean Diet: Rich in fruits, vegetables, whole grains, fish, and healthy fats (especially olive oil), this diet has been linked to a reduced risk of neurodegenerative diseases like Alzheimer's. Studies suggest it promotes better cognitive aging due to its anti-inflammatory properties.

- DASH Diet: Originally designed to combat hypertension, the DASH (Dietary Approaches to Stop Hypertension) diet emphasizes fruits, vegetables, whole grains, and low-fat dairy while minimizing saturated fats. Research indicates it may also support cognitive function by reducing inflammation.

- MIND Diet: A hybrid of the Mediterranean and DASH diets, the MIND (Mediterranean-DASH Intervention for Neurodegenerative Delay) diet focuses on brain-healthy foods such as leafy greens, nuts, berries, and fish. Studies have shown that adherence to this diet can slow cognitive decline significantly.

Essential Nutrients for Cognitive Function

Certain nutrients are particularly beneficial for brain health:

- **Omega-3 Fatty Acids**: Found in fatty fish (like salmon), walnuts, and flaxseeds, omega-3s are crucial for building and repairing brain cells. They have been linked to improved memory and overall cognitive function.

- **Antioxidants**: Foods rich in antioxidants—such as berries—help reduce oxidative stress in the brain. Flavonoids found in berries are associated with improved memory performance.

- **Vitamins and Minerals**: Leafy greens are high in nutrients like vitamin K, lutein, folate, and beta carotene—all of which have been shown to help slow cognitive decline.

Implications for Mental Health

The implications of these findings extend beyond cognitive function; they also encompass mental health. Diets high in processed foods and sugars have been linked to increased risks of depression and anxiety disorders. Conversely, a balanced diet rich in whole foods can enhance mood and emotional well-being.

Dr. James Ellison from the Swank Center for Memory Care emphasizes that "the foods we eat play a critical role in regulating everything in our bodies," underscoring the importance of dietary choices not just for physical health but also for mental resilience.

Summary

The evidence clearly supports the notion that a well-rounded diet is fundamental for maintaining brain health throughout life. By prioritizing balanced eating patterns rich in essential nutrients—such as those found in the Mediterranean or MIND diets—individuals can potentially reduce their risk of cognitive decline and enhance their overall mental well-being. As researchers continue to explore these connections, it becomes increasingly clear that our dietary choices hold significant power over our cognitive futures.

CHAPTER 12: EXERCISE AND BRAIN HEALTH

The connection between exercise and brain health has become a focal point of scientific research, revealing profound implications for cognitive function, memory, and overall mental well-being. This chapter examines how various forms of physical activity enhance brain health, supported by recent studies and expert commentary.

The Cognitive Benefits of Exercise

Research consistently demonstrates that regular physical activity is associated with improvements in cognitive function. A study from the University of British Columbia found that aerobic exercise—activities that elevate heart rate—can increase the size of the hippocampus, a brain region critical for memory and learning. Dr. Scott McGinnis, a neurologist at Harvard Medical School, emphasizes that "engaging in a program of regular exercise of moderate intensity over six months or a year is associated with an increase in the volume of selected brain regions," highlighting the long-term benefits of sustained physical activity.

Moreover, exercise has been shown to enhance executive functions such as attention and working memory. A study published in Scientific Reports indicated that participants who walked in natural outdoor environments performed significantly better on cognitive tasks than those who walked indoors. This suggests that not only does exercise improve cognitive performance, but the environment in which it occurs can amplify these benefits.

Mechanisms behind Exercise-Induced Cognitive Enhancements

The mechanisms through which exercise benefits the brain are manifold:

- **Increased Blood Flow**: Physical activity boosts blood circulation to the brain, delivering essential nutrients and oxygen necessary for optimal brain function. This increased blood flow is crucial since the brain has high metabolic demands.

- **Neurotrophic Factors**: Exercise stimulates the production of brain-derived neurotrophic factor (BDNF), a protein that supports neuron growth and survival. Higher levels of BDNF are linked to improved memory and learning capabilities.

- **Neuroplasticity:** Regular physical activity promotes neuroplasticity—the brain's ability to form new neural connections throughout life. This adaptability is vital for learning and memory retention.

- Stress Reduction: Exercise can mitigate stress by reducing the number of stress receptors in the hippocampus, thereby lessening the impact of stress hormones on cognitive function. The phenomenon known as "runner's high," characterized by endorphin release during exercise, further contributes to improved mood and reduced anxiety.

Types of Exercise Beneficial for Brain Health

While aerobic exercises like walking, running, or cycling are widely studied for their cognitive benefits, other forms of physical activity also play a role:

- Tai Chi: This martial art combines slow movements with mental focus and has been shown to enhance cognitive function in older adults, particularly in executive functions such as planning and problem-solving.

- Strength Training: Although primarily associated with physical fitness, resistance training may also contribute to cognitive health by improving overall body composition and metabolic health.

Outdoor vs. Indoor Exercise

Interestingly, the setting of exercise can influence its effectiveness on cognition. Studies indicate that outdoor exercise may provide additional cognitive benefits compared to indoor workouts. For instance, as shown in the studies mentioned above, participants who engaged in outdoor walking demonstrated greater enhancements in attention and working memory than those who exercised indoors. This aligns with Attention Restoration Theory, which posits that natural environments help restore depleted cognitive resources.

Summary

The evidence supporting the positive impact of exercise on brain health is robust and growing. Regular physical activity not only enhances cognitive functions but also fosters emotional well-being through various biological mechanisms. As Dr. Bonner-Jackson notes, "even in people who are at risk for development of Alzheimer's or other dementias, (exercise) can stave off decline in some cases for many years". Therefore, incorporating regular exercise into daily routines is essential for maintaining cognitive health throughout life.

CHAPTER 13: SLEEP AND BRAIN HEALTH

Sleep is a fundamental aspect of human health, playing an essential role in cognitive function, emotional regulation, and overall brain health. Recent research underscores the importance of sleep quality and duration in maintaining optimal brain function and preventing neurodegenerative diseases. This chapter explores how sleep affects brain health, supported by recent studies and expert insights.

The Impact of Sleep on Cognitive Function

Numerous studies have established a clear link between sleep and cognitive performance. According to research published in Scientific Reports, poor sleep—defined as less than six hours or more than nine hours per night—was associated with lower brain health indicators in midlife adults. The study analyzed data from nearly 30,000 participants and found that both short and long sleep durations correlated with reduced gray matter volume and cognitive impairments, including memory deficits and slower reaction times.

Dr. Clocchiatti-Tuozzo from Yale School of Medicine noted that "sleeping too much or too little is significantly correlated with neuroimaging markers of poor brain health," emphasizing that suboptimal sleep can lead to silent brain injuries that increase the risk of stroke and dementia later in life. This finding highlights the critical role that sleep plays not just in immediate cognitive function but also in long-term brain health.

Mechanisms behind Sleep's Influence on the Brain

The relationship between sleep and brain health is supported by several biological mechanisms:

- Memory Consolidation: During sleep, particularly during REM (rapid eye movement) sleep, the brain consolidates memories and processes information acquired throughout the day. This phase is essential for learning new skills and retaining information.

- Waste Clearance: Sleep facilitates the removal of waste products from brain cells, including amyloid plaques associated with Alzheimer's disease. The glymphatic system, which becomes more active during sleep, helps clear these toxins from the brain.

- Neuroplasticity: Adequate sleep is vital for neuroplasticity—the brain's ability to adapt and reorganize itself. Insufficient sleep impairs this process, *making it difficult to learn new information or remember previously learned material.*

Optimal Sleep Duration

Structure of sleep

- Non-rapid eye movement sleep (NREM)
- Rapid eye movement sleep (REM)

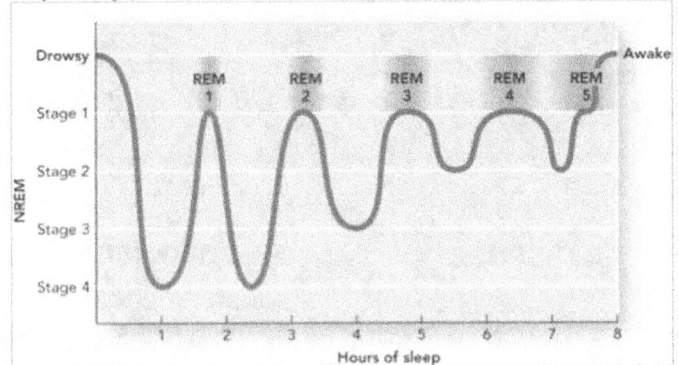

Research indicates that there is an optimal range for sleep duration that supports brain health. The American Heart Association recommends 7 to 9 hours of sleep per night for adults. Studies have shown that individuals who consistently fall outside this range—either sleeping less than 6 hours or more than 9 hours—exhibit poorer cognitive performance and lower brain volumes.

A U-shaped relationship has been observed between sleep duration and cognitive outcomes; both insufficient and excessive sleep are linked to negative effects on brain structure and function. For instance, individuals sleeping more than 9 hours per night were found to have approximately 0.75% less gray matter compared to those sleeping within the optimal range.

The Role of Sleep Disorders

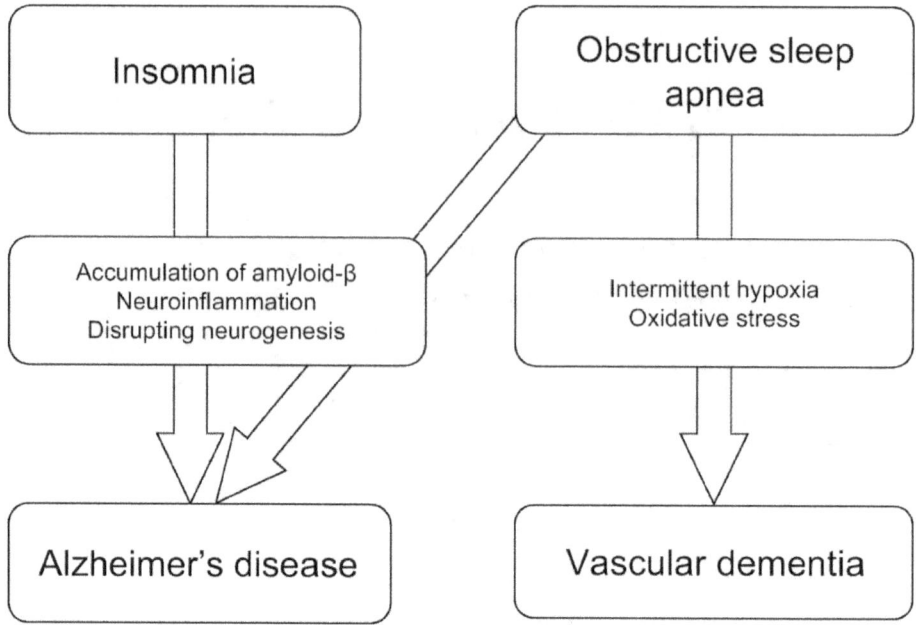

Sleep disorders such as insomnia or sleep apnea can significantly impact brain health. These conditions not only disrupt normal sleep patterns but also contribute to increased risks of cognitive decline and mood disorders. Research indicates that addressing these disorders can lead to improvements in cognitive function and overall mental health. Dr. McGinnis emphasizes that "treating sleep disorders represents a potential target for early intervention strategies aimed at improving brain health" as these conditions are often modifiable risk factors.

Summary

The evidence linking sleep to brain health is compelling. Quality sleep is essential for cognitive function, memory consolidation, emotional regulation, and the removal of neurotoxic waste from the brain. As researchers continue to explore this complex relationship, it becomes increasingly clear that prioritizing good sleep hygiene is crucial for maintaining optimal brain health throughout life. As Dr. Clocchiatti-Tuozzo aptly puts it, "sleep is a prime pillar of brain health," underscoring its importance as a modifiable risk factor for cognitive decline in later years.

CHAPTER 14: GENETICS OF DEMENTIA: RISK FACTORS AND BIOMARKERS

The genetic underpinnings of dementia are complex and multifaceted. While not all cases of dementia are hereditary, certain genetic factors significantly increase the risk of developing conditions like Alzheimer's disease (AD). This chapter explores the key genetic risk factors associated with dementia, including familial and sporadic forms, and highlights the biomarkers that may aid in early diagnosis.

Genetic Risk Factors

Familial Alzheimer's Disease

Familial Alzheimer's disease (FAD) is a rare, inherited form of AD that typically manifests at an earlier age, often in individuals in their 40s or 50s. FAD is primarily linked to mutations in three genes:

- Amyloid Precursor Protein (APP): Located on chromosome 21, mutations in this gene lead to abnormal processing of amyloid-beta (Aβ), promoting plaque formation.

- Presenilin 1 (PSEN1): Found on chromosome 14, PSEN1 mutations are the most common cause of early-onset familial AD.

- Presenilin 2 (PSEN2): Located on chromosome 1, mutations in this gene also contribute to familial forms of AD.

Individuals carrying these mutations have a near-certain likelihood of developing dementia, making genetic testing crucial for at-risk families (Queensland Brain Institute).

Late-Onset Alzheimer's Disease

In contrast, late-onset Alzheimer's disease is more common and typically occurs after the age of 65. The primary genetic risk factor for late-onset AD is the presence of the Apolipoprotein E (ApoE) gene variant known as ApoE4. Research indicates that individuals with one copy of ApoE4 are approximately three times more likely to develop AD, while those with two copies face a risk increase of five to eight times (Queensland Brain Institute; JAMA Neurology).

Despite its association with increased risk, it is important to note that not all individuals with ApoE4 develop AD. "Half or more of people with Alzheimer's disease have at least one copy of the ApoE4 gene—but while it means that the chances are higher of developing the disease, it is not inevitable" (Dementia Australia).

Other Genetic Contributions

Beyond APP, PSEN1, PSEN2, and ApoE4, several other genes have been implicated in increasing the risk for dementia. These include genes associated with inflammation and lipid metabolism. However, their contribution remains relatively minor compared to the aforementioned genes. For example, about 10% of cases of dementia with Lewy bodies and 10-15% of frontotemporal dementia cases exhibit hereditary patterns (Queensland Brain Institute).

Biomarkers for Early Diagnosis

Identifying genetic risk factors can aid in early diagnosis and intervention. Biomarkers such as Aβ levels in cerebrospinal fluid (CSF), neuroimaging findings indicating tau pathology, and genetic testing for known risk alleles can provide valuable insights into an individual's risk profile.

Recent studies suggest that "the combination of genetic testing and biomarker analysis can enhance diagnostic accuracy and enable earlier therapeutic interventions" (Griciuc & Tanzi, 2021). Early detection is crucial for managing symptoms and planning care effectively.

Summary

Understanding the genetic landscape of dementia provides essential insights into its etiology and potential interventions. While genetic factors can significantly influence the risk of developing conditions like Alzheimer's disease, they do not determine fate. As we continue our exploration in this book, we will discuss how lifestyle choices can further impact brain health and potentially mitigate genetic risks.

"Genetic risk factors offer a window into understanding the

complex interplay between heredity and environmental influences on dementia" (Griciuc & Tanzi, 2021).

CHAPTER 15: THE IMPACT OF LIFESTYLE ON BRAIN HEALTH

Lifestyle choices significantly influence brain health and can either mitigate or exacerbate the risk of developing dementia. This chapter examines the key lifestyle factors associated with cognitive decline, drawing on recent research to highlight actionable strategies for maintaining brain health throughout life.

Physical Activity

Regular physical activity is one of the most effective ways to preserve cognitive function. Studies have shown that adults who engage in regular exercise are less prone to memory loss later in life. For instance, a study published in the Journal of Alzheimer's Disease found that "physical activity can reduce the risk of dementia by up to 30-40% in older adults" (Colcombe et al., 2006).

Exercise promotes cardiovascular health, which is crucial for maintaining optimal blood flow to the brain. The FINGER study demonstrated that a two-year lifestyle intervention targeting physical activity, diet, and cognitive training led to improved cognitive function in at-risk older individuals (Ngandu et al., 2015).

Nutrition

Diet plays a vital role in brain health. The Mediterranean diet, rich in fruits, vegetables, whole grains, and healthy fats, has been associated with a reduced risk of cognitive decline. Research indicates that adherence to this dietary pattern can lower the risk of Alzheimer's disease (MIND diet) and improve overall cognitive function (Sofi et al., 2010).

Foods rich in antioxidants, such as berries and leafy greens, as well as omega-3 fatty acids found in fish, are particularly beneficial. According to the Alzheimer's Association, "healthy eating habits can help reduce the risk of cognitive decline" (Alzheimer's Association).

Mental Well-being

Mental health is closely linked to brain health. Chronic stress, anxiety, and depression can accelerate cognitive decline. A survey conducted by the Norwegian Institute of Public Health revealed that "99% of respondents associated Alzheimer's disease and dementia with mental health" (Budin-Ljøsne et al., 2022).

Engaging in mindfulness practices, such as meditation and yoga, can help manage stress levels and improve emotional well-being. Furthermore, social interactions are crucial; individuals with strong community ties tend to experience better mental health outcomes and reduced dementia risk (AARP Global Council on Brain Health).

Sleep Quality

Quality sleep is essential for cognitive function. Poor sleep patterns have been linked to an increased risk of developing mild cognitive impairment and dementia. Research indicates that "sleep disturbances can lead to accelerated cognitive decline" (Xie et al., 2019).

Establishing a consistent sleep routine and creating a conducive sleep environment can enhance sleep quality. Limiting screen time before bed and managing caffeine intake are practical steps individuals can take to improve their sleep hygiene.

Avoiding Harmful Substances

As earlier mentioned, substance use, including alcohol and tobacco, poses significant risks to brain health. Studies suggest that "quitting smoking can lower the risk of cognitive decline back to levels similar to those who have never smoked" (Alzheimer's Association). Additionally, excessive alcohol consumption is associated with an increased risk of dementia.

Social Determinants

Social determinants such as socioeconomic status and education level also influence lifestyle choices and brain health. Individuals with higher education levels tend to engage more in activities that promote brain health (Deckers et al., 2022). Addressing these social factors is crucial for implementing effective public health strategies aimed at reducing dementia risk.

Summary

Lifestyle choices play a critical role in shaping brain health and mitigating the risk of dementia. By adopting healthy habits—such as regular physical activity, a balanced diet, good sleep hygiene, mental well-being practices, and avoiding harmful substances—individuals can significantly impact their cognitive longevity. As we move forward in this book, we will explore current research and future directions in treatment options for dementia.

"Lifestyle changes have a substantial impact on brain health; therefore, prevention should always be the primary treatment tool" (Deckers et al., 2022).

CHAPTER 16: THE EMOTIONAL IMPACT OF DEMENTIA

The diagnosis of dementia can evoke a profound emotional response, not only in the individual receiving the diagnosis but also in their family and caregivers. Understanding these emotional reactions is crucial for providing effective support and fostering resilience throughout the caregiving journey. This chapter explores the range of emotions experienced by those diagnosed with dementia, the implications for caregivers, and strategies for managing these emotional challenges.

Emotional Responses to Diagnosis

Receiving a dementia diagnosis can trigger a complex array of emotions. Common reactions include:

- Shock and Disbelief: Many individuals experience initial disbelief, particularly if the diagnosis comes unexpectedly. This reaction can be compounded in cases of younger-onset dementia, where symptoms appear before age 65 (Dementia UK).

- Grief and Loss: A diagnosis often leads to feelings of grief as individuals come to terms with the loss of their cognitive abilities and the future they envisioned. This grief can manifest as sadness, anger, or frustration (Alzheimer's Society).

- Anxiety and Fear: Concerns about the progression of the disease, loss of independence, and the impact on loved ones can lead to significant anxiety. Individuals may fear moments of confusion or forgetfulness, which can exacerbate feelings of helplessness (Burns & Iliffe, 2009).

- Relief: Conversely, some individuals may feel relief upon receiving a diagnosis, as it provides an explanation for their symptoms and allows them to seek appropriate support (Dementia UK).

These emotional responses are not static; individuals may move between different feelings as they adjust to their new reality. Understanding this emotional landscape is essential for caregivers who play a vital role in supporting their loved ones through this transition.

The Impact on Caregivers

Caregivers also experience a range of emotions when a loved one is diagnosed with dementia. They may feel:

- Overwhelmed: The responsibilities associated with caregiving can lead to feelings of being overwhelmed, particularly when navigating complex medical and emotional needs (McLellan et al., 2008).

- Guilt: Caregivers may grapple with guilt about their loved one's condition or their ability to provide adequate support.

- Sadness and Grief: Witnessing the decline in a loved one's cognitive abilities can evoke profound sadness and anticipatory grief (Kessing et al., 2010).

- Frustration: Caregivers may feel frustrated by communication challenges or behavioral changes in their loved ones, which can lead to conflicts or misunderstandings.

Recognizing these emotions is critical for caregivers to ensure they seek support for themselves while providing compassionate care.

Managing Emotional Challenges

1. Encouraging Open Communication: Creating an environment where emotions can be openly discussed is vital. Encouraging individuals with dementia to express their feelings helps validate their experiences and fosters connection.

2. Seeking Professional Support: Therapy or counseling can be beneficial for both individuals with dementia and caregivers. Professional support provides a safe space to process emotions and develop coping strategies (Dementia UK).

3. Utilizing Support Groups: Joining support groups allows caregivers and individuals with dementia to share experiences with others facing similar challenges. These groups offer emotional validation and practical advice (Cattan et al., 2005).

4. Practicing Self-Care: Caregivers must prioritize self-care to manage stress effectively. Engaging in activities that promote physical and emotional well-being—such as exercise, hobbies, or mindfulness—can help mitigate caregiver burnout.

5. Educating about Dementia: Understanding the nature of dementia can help both patients and caregivers contextualize emotional responses. Education about the condition fosters empathy and patience in navigating difficult moments (Alzheimer's Association).

Summary

The emotional impact of a dementia diagnosis is profound and multifaceted, affecting both individuals with dementia and their caregivers. By recognizing and validating these emotions, we can foster resilience and connection during this challenging journey. As noted by Shara, a caregiver reflecting on her experience, "Understanding why we feel what we feel helps us cope better; it allows us to be more present for our loved ones."

By addressing the emotional dimensions of dementia care, we lay the foundation for compassionate support that honors both the individual living with dementia and those who care for them. In doing so, we create an environment conducive to healing, understanding, and ultimately reclaiming memories amidst the challenges posed by this condition.

CHAPTER 17: CARING FOR DEMENTIA PATIENTS: A BIOCHEMICAL APPROACH

Caring for individuals with dementia requires a comprehensive understanding of both the biochemical aspects of the disease and the psychosocial needs of patients. This chapter explores strategies for providing effective, person-centered care that integrates biomedical knowledge with psychosocial support, enhancing the quality of life for those affected by dementia.

Understanding Person-Centered Care

Person-centered care (PCC) is an approach that prioritizes the individual needs, preferences, and values of dementia patients. It emphasizes understanding the person behind the diagnosis, fostering a therapeutic relationship that respects their dignity and autonomy. According to Nicholson (2020), "Combining a bio-psychosocial approach with person-centered care principles allows people with dementia to have their personal, social, and emotional needs met".

The Bio-Psychosocial Model

The bio-psychosocial model integrates biological, psychological, and social factors affecting health. This holistic approach is essential in dementia care, as it acknowledges that cognitive decline is not solely a biomedical issue but also influenced by social interactions and emotional well-being. Research shows that "effective interventions often require a combination of biomedical and psychosocial perspectives" (Livingston et al., 2017).

Strategies for Effective Care

1. Tailored Interventions

Understanding the specific biochemical changes associated with different types of dementia can inform tailored interventions. For instance, cognitive stimulation therapy—structured activities like singing and baking—has been shown to preserve cognitive abilities in individuals with mild-to-moderate dementia (Knapp et al., 2006). These activities not only engage patients cognitively but also provide social interaction, which is vital for emotional health.

2. Medication Management

While non-pharmacological interventions are crucial, pharmacological treatments also play a role in managing symptoms. Acetylcholinesterase inhibitors (AChEIs) like donepezil and rivastigmine can help improve cholinergic transmission in patients with Alzheimer's disease (NICE). However, healthcare providers must monitor these medications closely to manage potential side effects effectively.

3. Creating Supportive Environments

A supportive environment can significantly impact the well-being of dementia patients. Modifying living spaces to reduce confusion—such as using clear signage and maintaining familiar routines—can help ease anxiety and enhance independence. Research indicates that "environmental modifications can lead to improved outcomes in behavioral symptoms" (Gove et al., 2018).

4. Engaging Families and Caregivers

Involving families and caregivers in the care process is essential. Education about the biochemical aspects of dementia can empower caregivers to understand behaviors better and respond appropriately. As noted by Quinn et al. (2017), "Developing a therapeutic relationship through education can support caregivers in managing daily challenges".

Addressing Behavioral Symptoms

Behavioral symptoms are common in dementia patients and can be challenging to manage. Understanding the underlying biochemical changes can help caregivers respond effectively:

- Aggression: Often linked to frustration or unmet needs, caregivers should assess environmental triggers and adjust accordingly.
- Anxiety: May stem from confusion; maintaining a calm environment can alleviate distress.
- Depression: Recognizing signs of depression is crucial; psychosocial interventions such as counseling or support

groups can be beneficial.

Summary

Caring for individuals with dementia requires a nuanced understanding that combines biochemical knowledge with compassionate, person-centered approaches. By integrating biomedical insights into daily care practices, healthcare providers can enhance the quality of life for patients while also supporting their families. As we continue our exploration in this book, we will delve into current research on treatment options and future directions in dementia care.

"A combined approach can help with effective symptom management, predicting disease progression, and planning for care" (Gove et al., 2018).

CHAPTER 18: EFFECTIVE COMMUNICATION TECHNIQUES

Effective communication is a cornerstone of quality dementia care. As cognitive abilities decline, individuals with dementia may struggle to express themselves and understand others, leading to frustration and misunderstandings. This chapter explores essential communication techniques that caregivers can employ to enhance interactions with individuals living with dementia, fostering connection and understanding.

Understanding Communication Challenges

Individuals with dementia often face significant communication difficulties due to cognitive and linguistic decline. Common challenges include:

- Word-Finding Difficulties: Individuals may struggle to recall words or phrases, leading to pauses or incomplete sentences. This can result in frustration for both the individual and the caregiver (Downs & Bowers, 2014).

- Reduced Comprehension: As dementia progresses, the ability to comprehend complex sentences diminishes. Individuals may find it challenging to follow conversations or instructions (Egan et al., 2010).

- Behavioral Changes: Changes in mood or behavior can further complicate communication. Anxiety, confusion, or agitation may hinder effective interactions (Burns & Iliffe, 2009).

Recognizing these challenges is the first step in developing effective communication strategies that can facilitate meaningful exchanges.

Key Communication Techniques

1. Use Simple Language: Employ short, clear sentences and avoid jargon. Research suggests that using simple language helps individuals with dementia better understand what is being communicated (Alzheimer's Society, 2016). For example:

    - Instead of saying, "Would you like to join us for dinner at the restaurant later?" say, "Dinner is ready. Would you like to eat now?"

2. One Idea at a Time: Present one question or idea at a time to avoid overwhelming the individual. This technique allows for clearer understanding and reduces confusion (Egan et al., 2010).

3. Maintain Eye Contact: Establishing eye contact helps create a connection and shows that you are engaged in the conversation. It also allows individuals with dementia to focus on your facial expressions and body language (Alzheimer's Society, 2016).

4. Use Non-Verbal Communication: Non-verbal cues such as gestures, facial expressions, and touch can enhance understanding and convey emotions when verbal communication is challenging. For example, smiling while offering assistance can create a positive atmosphere (Downs & Bowers, 2014).

5. Eliminate Distractions: Reduce background noise and visual distractions during conversations. A calm environment promotes better focus and comprehension (Egan et al., 2010).

6. Incorporate Meaningful Objects: Use photographs, objects, or memory aids that hold significance for the individual. These items can spark memories and facilitate conversation by providing context (Kindell et al., 2016).

7. Practice Patience: Allow individuals time to process information and respond without rushing them. Patience conveys respect and understanding, fostering a supportive environment for communication (Burns & Iliffe, 2009).

8. Encourage Expression: Create opportunities for individuals to express their feelings or thoughts through various means —verbal communication, art, music, or writing—encouraging them to find ways that resonate with them (Smebye et al., 2012).

Training Caregivers in Communication Skills

Training programs focused on enhancing communication skills for caregivers have shown promising results in improving interactions with individuals living with dementia. For instance:

- The TRACED program integrates empirically informed approaches that address cognitive limitations while fostering relational connections between caregivers and individuals with dementia (Ojha et al., 2020).

- Communication skills training has been linked to improved quality of life for patients with dementia by increasing positive interactions in care settings (Alm et al., 2004; Egan et al., 2010).

These training programs equip caregivers with practical tools and techniques necessary for effective communication, ultimately enhancing the caregiving experience.

Summary

Effective communication is vital in supporting individuals living with dementia as they navigate the complexities of their condition. By employing strategies such as using simple language, maintaining eye contact, incorporating meaningful objects, and practicing patience, caregivers can foster meaningful connections that enhance the quality of life for those they support.

As Dr. David Knopman emphasizes, "Communication is not just about words; it's about connection." By prioritizing effective communication techniques, we honor the dignity of individuals living with dementia and ensure their voices are heard amidst the challenges they face.

CHAPTER 19: DAILY LIVING AND CARE STRATEGIES

As dementia progresses, individuals may face increasing challenges in daily living, necessitating tailored care strategies to enhance their quality of life. This chapter explores practical approaches to daily living that can help individuals with dementia maintain independence, dignity, and engagement in meaningful activities. By implementing effective care strategies, caregivers can create supportive environments that promote well-being.

Creating a Safe and Supportive Environment

A safe environment is crucial for individuals with dementia. Modifications can significantly reduce the risk of accidents and enhance comfort:

- Declutter Living Spaces: Reducing clutter minimizes confusion and helps individuals navigate their surroundings more easily. A tidy environment can also decrease anxiety levels (Mayo Clinic, 2024).

- Use Visual Cues: Labeling rooms and important items with

clear signs can aid memory and orientation. For instance, placing labels on bathroom doors or kitchen cabinets can help individuals locate essential areas more easily (Alzheimer's Society, 2016).

- Ensure Adequate Lighting: Good lighting is essential to prevent disorientation and falls. Night lights in hallways and bedrooms can provide reassurance during nighttime (Mayo Clinic, 2024).

- Create a Routine: Establishing a consistent daily routine provides structure and predictability, which can be comforting for individuals with dementia. Regular schedules for meals, activities, and bedtime help reduce anxiety associated with uncertainty (Alzheimer's Association, 2021).

Engaging in Meaningful Activities

Engagement in meaningful activities is vital for cognitive stimulation and emotional well-being. Caregivers should consider the following strategies:

1. **Tailor Activities to Interests:** Identify hobbies or interests that the individual enjoyed before their diagnosis. *Activities such as gardening, painting, or listening to music can evoke positive memories and foster engagement (Mayo Clinic, 2024).*

2. **Incorporate Physical Activity:** Regular physical activity has been shown to slow cognitive decline and improve mood. Simple exercises like walking or dancing can be enjoyable and beneficial for both physical health and emotional well-being (Lancet Commission on Dementia Prevention, 2020).

3. **Use Reminiscence Therapy**: Engaging individuals in reminiscence therapy—discussing past experiences using

photographs or familiar objects—can stimulate memory recall and enhance emotional connections (Simmons-Stern et al., 2010).

4. **Encourage Social Interaction:** Facilitating social interactions with friends or family members helps combat feelings of isolation. Group activities or community programs designed for individuals with dementia can promote social engagement (Cattan et al., 2005).

Supporting Daily Living Tasks

As dementia progresses, individuals may require assistance with daily living tasks. Caregivers should approach these tasks with sensitivity and respect:

- Promote Independence: Encourage individuals to perform tasks they are still capable of completing independently. This approach fosters a sense of autonomy and self-worth (Mayo Clinic, 2024).

- Break Tasks into Steps: Simplifying tasks by breaking them into smaller steps can make them more manageable. For example, when preparing a meal, caregivers can guide individuals through each step rather than overwhelming them with the entire process at once (Egan et al., 2010).

- Use Adaptive Equipment: Consider using adaptive tools designed to assist with daily tasks. For instance, utensils with larger grips or non-slip mats can help individuals maintain independence while reducing frustration (Alzheimer's Society, 2016).

Establishing Nighttime Routines

Behavioral changes often worsen at night—a phenomenon known as "sundowning." Establishing calming nighttime routines can help mitigate these issues:

- Create a Calming Environment: Limit noise from televisions or other distractions during the evening hours. A quiet atmosphere promotes relaxation before bedtime (Mayo Clinic, 2024).

- Implement a Consistent Bedtime Routine: Engage in calming activities such as reading or listening to soft music before bed to signal that it is time to wind down.

- Monitor Diet and Caffeine Intake: Reducing caffeine consumption later in the day can improve sleep quality. Additionally, establishing regular meal times helps regulate sleep patterns (Mayo Clinic, 2024).

Summary

Implementing effective daily living strategies is essential for enhancing the quality of life for individuals living with dementia. By creating safe environments, engaging in meaningful activities, supporting daily tasks, and establishing calming nighttime routines, caregivers can foster independence while providing compassionate care.

As Dr. David Knopman emphasizes: "Empowering individuals with dementia through tailored support not only enhances their well-being but also enriches the caregiving experience." By prioritizing these strategies, we honor the dignity of those we care for while navigating the complexities of dementia together.

CHAPTER 20: EARLY SIGNS AND SYMPTOMS OF DEMENTIA IN WOMEN

Dementia is a complex syndrome that manifests through various cognitive and behavioral changes. Research indicates that women may experience distinct early signs and symptoms, which can sometimes be subtle and easily overlooked. The following are the key early indicators to watch for:

1. Memory Loss

One of the most common early signs of dementia is memory lapses, particularly concerning recent events. Women may forget familiar words or misplace everyday items. As noted by Medical News Today, "Mild forgetfulness, changes to perception or the way we speak can be early indications that something is wrong". This can lead to frustration and anxiety for both the individual and their loved ones.

2. Confusion and Disorientation

Women may experience confusion in familiar settings, such as getting lost while driving or forgetting where they are. The

World Health Organization states that early symptoms include "getting lost when walking or driving" and "being confused, even in familiar places". This disorientation can be particularly distressing and may go unnoticed until it becomes more pronounced.

3. Communication Difficulties

Difficulty finding the right words or following conversations is another early symptom. According to Healthline, individuals may struggle to express their thoughts clearly or may stop mid-sentence, unsure of how to continue . This can make social interactions increasingly challenging.

4. Changes in Mood and Behavior

Emotional changes often occur before cognitive decline becomes apparent. Women may exhibit mood swings, increased anxiety, or withdrawal from social activities they once enjoyed. The Alzheimer's Research UK highlights that "low mood and anxiety are common early symptoms" . These emotional shifts can be mistaken for normal aging or stress.

5. Apathy and Loss of Initiative

A noticeable decline in interest in previously enjoyed activities is common in the early stages of dementia. Women may become apathetic about hobbies or social interactions, leading to isolation. Medical News Today notes that "individuals may become moody or withdrawn, especially in socially or mentally challenging situations" .

6. Difficulty with Problem-Solving

Women may find it increasingly challenging to complete familiar tasks or make decisions. This could manifest as trouble managing finances or following a recipe. The Better Health

Channel emphasizes that "a subtle shift in the ability to complete everyday tasks is another possible early indicator of dementia".

7. Behavioral Changes

Changes in personality and behavior can also signal early dementia. Women might become more suspicious or exhibit compulsive behaviors, such as hand-wringing or tissue shredding. The World Health Organization notes that common changes include "personality changes" and "withdrawal from work or social activities".

Summary

Recognizing these early signs of dementia in women is crucial for timely intervention and support. While these symptoms can overlap with other conditions such as depression or anxiety, persistent changes warrant a consultation with a healthcare professional for further evaluation. Early detection can lead to better management strategies that enhance quality of life and potentially slow disease progression.

"Dementia is a complex and multifaceted condition that requires early detection and proactive management".

CHAPTER 21: EARLY SIGNS AND SYMPTOMS OF DEMENTIA IN MEN

Dementia affects individuals differently, and while many symptoms are common across genders, men may exhibit specific early signs that can help in identifying the condition. Recognizing these symptoms early is crucial for timely intervention and management. The following are some key early indicators of dementia in men, supported by research and expert insights:

1. Memory Loss

Memory impairment is often one of the first noticeable signs of dementia. Men may experience subtle changes in their short-term memory, such as forgetting recent events or misplacing items. According to the World Health Organization, "forgetting things or recent events" is a common early symptom of dementia, which can escalate to more significant memory issues over time.

2. Difficulty with Communication

Men may struggle with finding the right words or following conversations. This difficulty can manifest as pauses in speech or an inability to articulate thoughts clearly. Healthline notes that "difficulty finding the right words" is a prevalent early indicator of dementia, making conversations challenging for both the individual and their listeners.

3. Increased Confusion

Confusion about time and place is another early sign. Men may find themselves disoriented in familiar environments or forget what day it is. The NHS emphasizes that "being confused about time and place" is a typical symptom that can lead to increased anxiety and frustration.

4. Changes in Mood and Behavior

Emotional changes often occur before cognitive decline becomes apparent. Men may exhibit mood swings, increased irritability, or withdrawal from social activities they once enjoyed. The Alzheimer's Research UK highlights that "low mood and anxiety are common early symptoms," which can complicate diagnosis as these feelings may be mistaken for normal aging or stress.

5. Apathy and Loss of Initiative

A noticeable decline in interest in hobbies or social interactions can be an early warning sign. Men may become apathetic about activities they previously enjoyed, leading to isolation. Healthline mentions that "apathy is a common symptom of early dementia," indicating a lack of motivation to engage with others.

6. Difficulty Completing Familiar Tasks

Men may begin to struggle with routine tasks, such as managing finances or following a recipe. The Better Health Channel states that "a subtle shift in the ability to complete everyday tasks" can signal the onset of dementia. This difficulty may manifest as forgetting steps in a process or needing assistance with previously manageable activities.

7. Poor Judgment

Deterioration in decision-making abilities is another concerning sign. Men might make poor financial decisions or exhibit lapses in judgment regarding personal safety. The World Health Organization notes that "losing track of time" and having trouble making decisions are common early symptoms.

Summary

Recognizing these early signs of dementia in men is essential for facilitating timely intervention and support. While these symptoms can overlap with other conditions such as depression or anxiety, persistent changes warrant a consultation with a healthcare professional for further evaluation. Early detection can lead to better management strategies that enhance quality of life and potentially slow disease progression.

"Dementia's signs and symptoms are often mild and not easily spotted at first; however, awareness is key for timely intervention".

CHAPTER 22: TESTS FOR DIAGNOSING DEMENTIA

Diagnosing dementia involves a comprehensive assessment that combines medical history, cognitive evaluations, and various diagnostic tests. No single test can definitively diagnose dementia; rather, healthcare professionals use a combination of approaches to arrive at an accurate diagnosis.

1. Medical History and Personal Assessment

The diagnostic process often begins with a detailed medical history. Physicians will ask about the patient's symptoms, their progression, and any changes in memory or behavior. It is helpful to involve family members or close friends who can provide additional insights into the individual's cognitive decline. According to Mayo Clinic, "A health care professional must recognize the pattern of loss of skills and function" to diagnose dementia effectively.

2. Cognitive Testing

Cognitive tests are an essential component of the evaluation process. These tests assess various cognitive functions, including memory, problem-solving abilities, language skills, and attention. Commonly used screening tools include the Mini-

Mental State Examination (MMSE) and the Montreal Cognitive Assessment (MoCA). As noted by Healthdirect, "A doctor may use tests to check the person's cognitive or thinking functions".

3. Neuropsychological Testing

In cases where cognitive screening yields inconclusive results, neuropsychological testing may be employed. This more extensive testing can identify specific areas of cognitive impairment and help differentiate between types of dementia. The National Institutes of Health emphasizes that "neuropsychological tests sometimes show characteristic results for people with different types of dementia".

4. Neurological Examination

A thorough neurological examination assesses motor skills, sensory perception, coordination, and reflexes. This helps rule out other potential causes of cognitive decline, such as neurological disorders or physical impairments.

5. Brain Imaging

Imaging techniques like MRI (Magnetic Resonance Imaging), CT (Computed Tomography), and PET (Positron Emission Tomography) scans are essential for visualizing brain structure and function. These scans can help identify abnormalities such as tumors, strokes, or signs of neurodegeneration associated with Alzheimer's disease. The Alzheimer's Association states that "brain imaging can reveal tumors, evidence of strokes, or damage from severe head trauma".

6. Laboratory Tests

Blood tests are performed to rule out other conditions that may mimic dementia symptoms, such as vitamin deficiencies (e.g., vitamin B12), thyroid disorders, or infections. According to Mayo Clinic, "simple blood tests can detect physical problems that can affect brain function". In some cases, cerebrospinal fluid analysis may be conducted to check for biomarkers associated with Alzheimer's disease.

7. Psychiatric Evaluation

A psychiatric assessment may be necessary to identify any coexisting mental health conditions that could contribute to cognitive symptoms, such as depression or anxiety disorders. The Better Health Channel notes that "psychiatric assessment helps to identify treatable disorders".

Summary

The diagnosis of dementia is a multifaceted process that requires careful evaluation by healthcare professionals. By employing a combination of medical history assessment, cognitive testing, imaging studies, laboratory tests, and psychiatric evaluations, clinicians can accurately diagnose dementia and differentiate it from other conditions with similar symptoms. Early diagnosis is crucial for effective management and treatment planning.

"No single test can determine if a person is living with Alzheimer's or another dementia; physicians use diagnostic tools combined with medical history and other information".

CHAPTER 23: MANAGING BEHAVIORAL CHANGES

Behavioral changes in individuals with dementia can be one of the most challenging aspects of caregiving. These changes may manifest as agitation, aggression, wandering, or other unpredictable behaviors that can be distressing for both the individual and their caregivers. Understanding the underlying causes of these behaviors and implementing effective management strategies is essential for improving quality of life and fostering a supportive environment. This chapter explores common behavioral changes in dementia, their triggers, and practical approaches to managing them.

Common Behavioral Changes

Individuals with dementia often exhibit a range of behavioral changes, including:

- Agitation and Aggression: Individuals may become restless, irritable, or aggressive, often due to frustration or confusion. Research indicates that these behaviors are frequently triggered by unmet needs or environmental stressors (Burns & Iliffe, 2009).

- Wandering: Many individuals with dementia may wander aimlessly, which can pose safety risks. This behavior often stems from disorientation or the need for movement (Alzheimer's Association, 2021).

- Repetitive Questions or Actions: Individuals may ask the same questions repeatedly or perform the same actions multiple times, stemming from memory loss and confusion about their surroundings (Egan et al., 2010).

Understanding the Causes

Behavioral changes in dementia can result from various factors:

1. Cognitive Decline: As cognitive abilities deteriorate, individuals may struggle to process information or communicate effectively, leading to frustration and behavioral outbursts (Alzheimer's Society, 2016).

2. Environmental Triggers: Overstimulation from noise, unfamiliar surroundings, or even changes in routine can provoke agitation. A study found that a calm and familiar environment significantly reduces instances of challenging behavior (BMC Geriatrics, 2018).

3. Physical Discomfort: Pain or discomfort that goes unrecognized can lead to agitation. Caregivers should be vigilant in assessing for signs of pain or illness that may not be verbally communicated (Burns & Iliffe, 2009).

4. Emotional Factors: Feelings of fear, anxiety, or loneliness can exacerbate behavioral changes. Individuals with dementia may become anxious in unfamiliar situations or when they feel isolated (Kessing et al., 2010).

Strategies for Management

1. Identify Triggers: Caregivers should observe and document specific triggers that lead to behavioral changes. Identifying patterns can help anticipate and mitigate these behaviors effectively (Alzheimer's Association, 2021).

2. Maintain a Calm Environment: Creating a peaceful atmosphere by reducing noise and clutter can help soothe agitation. A calm demeanor from caregivers also contributes to a more relaxed environment (BMC Geriatrics, 2018).

3. Use Validation Techniques: Instead of correcting misconceptions or insisting on reality, validating feelings can help reduce frustration. For instance, if an individual believes they need to go home, acknowledging their feelings rather than arguing can provide comfort (Feil, 2012).

4. Engage in Meaningful Activities: Providing structured activities that align with the individual's interests can redirect attention and reduce negative behaviors. Activities such as music therapy or art can foster engagement and joy (Simmons-Stern et al., 2010).

5. Implement Routine: Establishing a consistent daily routine helps individuals feel secure and reduces anxiety associated with unpredictability (Alzheimer's Association, 2021).

6. Use Redirection Techniques: When faced with agitation or repetitive questioning, gently redirecting the individual's focus to another topic or activity can help diffuse tension.

7. Involve Professional Support: If behavioral changes become severe or unmanageable, seeking assistance from healthcare professionals specializing in dementia care may be necessary. They can provide additional strategies tailored to the individual's needs (BMC Geriatrics, 2018).

The Role of Caregiver Support

Caregivers must also prioritize their well-being when managing behavioral changes. Training programs focused on behavioral management strategies have been shown to reduce caregiver stress and improve care quality (Gitlin et al., 2006). Support groups provide an opportunity for caregivers to share experiences and coping strategies.

Summary

Managing behavioral changes in individuals with dementia requires a comprehensive understanding of underlying causes and effective strategies tailored to each person's needs. By employing techniques such as identifying triggers, maintaining calm environments, engaging in meaningful activities, and seeking professional support when necessary, caregivers can significantly improve the quality of life for those they support.

As Dr. David Knopman states: "Compassionate understanding of behavior is key to navigating the challenges of dementia care." By fostering empathy and implementing effective management strategies, caregivers can create an environment that honors the dignity of individuals living with dementia while enhancing their overall well-being.

CHAPTER 24: LEGAL AND FINANCIAL CONSIDERATIONS IN DEMENTIA CARE

Navigating the legal and financial aspects of dementia care is crucial for ensuring that individuals receive appropriate support and that their wishes are respected. This chapter outlines essential considerations, including advance care planning, power of attorney, and financial management, to help families prepare for the complexities associated with dementia.

Advance Care Planning (ACP)

Advance care planning is a proactive process that allows individuals to express their preferences for future medical treatment and care while they still have the capacity to do so. Research indicates that early discussions about advance care planning can significantly benefit both patients and families. A study found that engaging in ACP soon after a dementia diagnosis can be perceived positively, as it provides clarity regarding the individual's wishes (Dening et al., 2013).

Advance care planning encompasses several key components:

- Advance Directives: These legal documents allow individuals to specify their healthcare preferences in advance, including decisions about life-sustaining treatments and palliative care options. Having an advance directive in place can alleviate family stress during critical decision-making moments (Alzheimer's Society, 2021).

- Do Not Resuscitate (DNR) Orders: A DNR order specifies that an individual does not wish to receive cardiopulmonary resuscitation (CPR) in the event of cardiac arrest. Discussing this option with healthcare providers can ensure that the individual's wishes are honored.

- Regular Review: It is essential to review advance directives periodically, especially as the individual's condition progresses or their preferences change. Keeping communication open among family members and healthcare providers ensures everyone is aware of the individual's wishes.

Power of Attorney

Establishing a power of attorney (POA) is vital for ensuring that trusted individuals can make financial and healthcare decisions on behalf of someone with dementia when they can no longer do so. There are two main types of POA:

1. Durable Power of Attorney for Health Care: This designation allows appointed individuals to make medical decisions when the person is incapacitated. It is crucial to discuss preferences regarding medical treatments and end-of-life care with the designated agent.

2. Durable Power of Attorney for Finances: This allows

appointed agents to manage financial affairs, including paying bills, managing assets, and making investment decisions. Establishing a financial POA early can prevent complications later on (National Institute on Aging).

Research shows that having a POA in place reduces family conflict and stress during critical decision-making periods (Alzheimer's Association, 2021). Families who engage in these discussions early on report feeling more secure about their financial decisions related to dementia care.

Managing Finances

Financial management becomes increasingly complex as dementia progresses. Caregivers should consider the following strategies:

- Budgeting: Establishing a clear budget helps manage expenses related to care. This includes understanding costs associated with medications, therapy, home modifications, and potential long-term care facilities.

- Monitoring Accounts: Regularly reviewing bank statements can help detect unusual transactions or potential financial abuse. Individuals with dementia may become vulnerable to scams or exploitation, making vigilance essential (Alzheimer's Society, 2021).

- Utilizing Professional Help: Consulting with financial advisors who specialize in elder care can provide valuable guidance on managing assets and planning for future expenses. These professionals can assist families in navigating complex financial decisions related to long-term care.

Legal Rights and Resources

Individuals with dementia retain certain legal rights, including the right to make decisions about their care as long as they have the capacity. It is vital for caregivers to understand these rights and seek legal counsel if necessary. Resources such as local elder law attorneys or advocacy organizations can provide support in navigating legal challenges.

Additionally, many communities offer resources for families dealing with dementia, including:

- Support Groups: These groups provide emotional support and practical advice from others facing similar challenges.

- Educational Workshops: Local organizations often host workshops focused on legal and financial planning for families affected by dementia.

Summary

Addressing legal and financial considerations is essential for ensuring that individuals with dementia receive appropriate care aligned with their wishes. By engaging in advance care planning, establishing power of attorney, and managing finances proactively, families can alleviate stress and enhance the quality of life for their loved ones.

As Dr. David Knopman emphasizes, "Empowering families through knowledge of legal rights and options is key to navigating the complexities of dementia care." By prioritizing these considerations, we honor the dignity of individuals living with dementia while ensuring their voices are heard throughout the caregiving journey.

CHAPTER 25: STAGES OF DEMENTIA, LIFE EXPECTANCY, AND TREATMENT

Dementia is a progressive syndrome characterized by a decline in cognitive function, affecting memory, thinking, and behavior. Understanding the stages of dementia, life expectancy, and available treatments is crucial for patients, caregivers, and healthcare providers.

Stages of Dementia

Dementia is often classified into seven stages, which can be grouped into three main categories: early, middle, and late stages.

1. No Cognitive Decline (Stage 1): Individuals exhibit no symptoms and function normally.

2. Very Mild Cognitive Decline (Stage 2): Minor memory lapses occur, often dismissed as normal aging.

3. Mild Cognitive Decline (Stage 3): Family members may notice forgetfulness and confusion. This stage typically lasts about 2 to 7 years.

4. Moderate Cognitive Decline (Stage 4): Individuals struggle with recent events and complex tasks. This stage can last approximately 2 years.

5. Moderately Severe Cognitive Decline (Stage 5): Severe memory loss occurs; individuals may forget personal information and require assistance with daily activities. This stage usually lasts around 1.5 years.

6. Severe Cognitive Decline (Stage 6): Patients often forget names of close family members and experience significant personality changes. This stage generally lasts about 2.5 years.

7. Very Severe Cognitive Decline (Stage 7): Individuals lose the ability to speak or walk and require full-time care. This final stage lasts between 1.5 to 2.5 years.

As noted by BuzzRx, "The average duration of the seven stages of dementia varies widely among individuals," influenced by factors like overall health and the specific type of dementia diagnosed.

Life Expectancy

Life expectancy for individuals diagnosed with dementia varies depending on the type of dementia:

- Alzheimer's Disease: Average life expectancy is about 8 to 10 years after diagnosis.

- Vascular Dementia: Typically around 5 years, due to associated risks like stroke.

- Dementia with Lewy Bodies: Average life expectancy is approximately 6 years.

- Frontotemporal Dementia: Life expectancy ranges from 6 to 8 years.

According to Healthline, "People with Alzheimer's disease live an average of 4 to 8 years after diagnosis, but some may live as long as 20 years" depending on various health factors.

Treatment Options

Currently, there is no cure for dementia; however, several treatment options can help manage symptoms and improve quality of life:

1. Medications:

- Cholinesterase Inhibitors (e.g., Donepezil) are commonly prescribed for Alzheimer's disease to help improve cognitive function by increasing levels of acetylcholine in the brain.

- Memantine is another medication that may help moderate to severe Alzheimer's by regulating glutamate activity.

2. Non-Pharmacological Interventions:

- Cognitive stimulation therapy (CST) has shown effectiveness in improving cognitive function and quality of life for individuals in early to moderate stages of dementia.

- Engaging in physical activities can also slow cognitive decline and improve overall well-being.

3. Supportive Care:

- Providing a structured environment can help manage behavioral symptoms.

- Caregiver support programs are essential for helping families cope with the challenges associated with dementia care.

As highlighted by Healthline, "While there's no cure for dementia, treatments can help manage symptoms and improve quality of life" . Early diagnosis and intervention are crucial in managing the disease effectively.

Summary

Understanding the stages of dementia, life expectancy, and treatment options provides valuable insights for those affected by this condition. With appropriate care and support, individuals with dementia can maintain a better quality of life throughout their journey.

"Dementia progresses uniquely in each individual; awareness and proactive management are key".

CHAPTER 26: TREATMENT FOR LEWY BODY DEMENTIA

Lewy Body Dementia (LBD) is a progressive condition characterized by cognitive decline, visual hallucinations, and motor symptoms similar to Parkinson's disease. While there is currently no cure for LBD, various treatments can help manage symptoms and improve the quality of life for those affected.

1. Medications

While no drugs can halt the progression of LBD, several medications can alleviate specific symptoms:

- Acetylcholinesterase Inhibitors: Medications such as donepezil (Aricept) and rivastigmine (Exelon) are often prescribed to help improve cognitive function and manage hallucinations. These drugs work by increasing levels of acetylcholine, a neurotransmitter important for memory and learning. According to the NHS, "These medications can help reduce hallucinations, confusion, and sleepiness".

- Levodopa: This medication is primarily used to treat Parkinson's disease and can help with movement problems in LBD patients. However, it must be used cautiously, as it can exacerbate other symptoms like hallucinations.

- Antipsychotics: Medications such as quetiapine may be prescribed for severe behavioral issues but should be used with caution due to potential side effects, including worsening cognitive symptoms.

- Melatonin and Clonazepam: These can be effective for managing sleep disturbances common in LBD, particularly REM sleep behavior disorder.

2. Non-Pharmacological Interventions

In addition to medication, various therapies can support individuals with LBD:

- Physical Therapy: Helps improve mobility and balance, addressing movement-related symptoms.

- Occupational Therapy: Assists individuals in adapting their daily activities to maintain independence.

- Cognitive Stimulation Therapy: Engages patients in activities designed to enhance cognitive function and social interaction.

- Psychological Therapies: Counseling or psychotherapy can help address mood disorders such as depression and anxiety, which are common in individuals with LBD.

3. Supportive Care

A comprehensive care plan is essential for managing LBD effectively. This may include:

- Home Modifications: Making adjustments to the living environment to enhance safety and accessibility.

- Support Groups: Connecting with others facing similar challenges can provide emotional support and practical advice.

- Caregiver Support: Educating caregivers about the specific needs of individuals with LBD can help them provide better care and reduce their own stress.

Life Expectancy

The average life expectancy after a diagnosis of Lewy Body Dementia is typically around 5 to 7 years, although this can vary significantly among individuals. Some may live longer depending on their overall health and the management of symptoms.

Summary

While there is no cure for Lewy Body Dementia, a combination of medications, therapies, and supportive care can significantly improve the quality of life for those affected. Early diagnosis and a tailored treatment plan are crucial in managing this complex condition effectively.

"There's currently no cure for dementia with Lewy bodies, but there

are treatments that can help manage the symptoms".

CHAPTER 27: END-OF-LIFE CARE FOR INDIVIDUALS WITH DEMENTIA

As dementia progresses, individuals approach a stage where end-of-life care becomes a critical concern. This chapter explores the unique challenges associated with providing quality end-of-life care for individuals with dementia, emphasizing the importance of planning, communication, and person-centered approaches to ensure dignity and comfort during this sensitive time.

Understanding End-of-Life Care in Dementia

End-of-life care refers to the support and medical care given during the final phase of life, typically when an individual is considered to be in their last twelve months. For individuals with dementia, this care must be tailored to address their specific needs, as they may experience a range of physical, emotional, and cognitive challenges (World Health Organization).

Research indicates that individuals with dementia often

receive suboptimal end-of-life care compared to those with other terminal illnesses such as cancer. A study highlighted that people with advanced dementia frequently experience inadequate pain control, increased hospitalizations, and fewer palliative care interventions (BMC Geriatrics, 2018). This disparity underscores the need for improved frameworks and practices in dementia end-of-life care.

Key Components of Quality End-of-Life Care

1. Timely Recognition of End of Life: Early identification of when an individual is nearing the end of life is crucial for appropriate planning and intervention. Healthcare professionals must be trained to recognize signs indicating that an individual with dementia is approaching this stage (BMC Palliative Care, 2024).

2. Advance Care Planning (ACP): Engaging in advance care planning allows individuals and their families to discuss preferences for medical treatment and end-of-life care while the person still has decision-making capacity. Research shows that discussions about ACP can be beneficial when initiated early in the disease trajectory (Dening et al., 2013). Families often feel more secure knowing their loved one's wishes regarding interventions such as resuscitation or palliative care options.

3. Person-Centered Care: Providing person-centered care involves tailoring support to meet the unique needs and preferences of the individual. This approach emphasizes dignity, respect, and comfort. According to a study by the Australian Commission on Safety and Quality in Health Care, person-centered practices significantly improve the quality of life for individuals with dementia at the end of life (BMC Palliative Care, 2024).

4. Effective Communication: Open communication among healthcare providers, caregivers, and family members is vital for ensuring that everyone is aligned with the individual's wishes. Regular discussions about changing needs and preferences can help adjust care plans appropriately (Alzheimer's Society, 2021).

5. Coordinated Care: Coordination among healthcare providers is essential for delivering comprehensive end-of-life care. This includes collaboration between primary care physicians, specialists, palliative care teams, and community services to ensure continuity and quality of care (BMC Geriatrics, 2018).

Challenges in End-of-Life Care

Despite advancements in understanding end-of-life care for individuals with dementia, several challenges persist:

- Barriers to Accessing Palliative Care: Many individuals with dementia do not receive appropriate palliative or hospice services due to misconceptions about their prognosis or lack of awareness among healthcare providers regarding suitable interventions (KCL Policy Brief).

- Family Dynamics: Families may struggle with decision-making around end-of-life care due to emotional distress or differing opinions on treatment options. Providing education and support can help families navigate these difficult conversations (Dening et al., 2013).

- Cultural Considerations: Cultural beliefs and values play a significant role in how families approach end-of-life decisions. It is essential for caregivers to be sensitive to these factors when discussing treatment options and preferences.

Summary

Providing quality end-of-life care for individuals with dementia requires a comprehensive understanding of their unique needs and challenges. By prioritizing timely recognition of end-of-life stages, engaging in advance care planning, fostering person-centered approaches, ensuring effective communication, and coordinating care among providers, we can enhance the quality of life during this critical time. By implementing these principles into practice, caregivers can create an environment that honors the wishes of individuals living with dementia while providing them with comfort and support as they transition through this final phase of life.

CHAPTER 28: SEVENTY-SEVEN (77) FACTS ABOUT DEMENTIA

1. Definition: Dementia is an umbrella term for a range of cognitive impairments that interfere with daily life and independence.

2. Prevalence: Approximately 55 million people worldwide are living with dementia, a number expected to rise to 139 million by 2050.

3. Leading Cause of Death: Dementia is the second leading cause of death in Australia and the leading cause of death for women in that country.

4. Projected Growth: In Australia, the number of people living with dementia is expected to increase from 421,000 in 2024 to over 812,500 by 2054.

5. Younger Onset Dementia: Nearly 29,000 Australians are estimated to be living with younger onset dementia (diagnosed before age 65), projected to rise to over 41,000 by 2054.

6. Global Impact: One in three people born today in the UK will develop dementia in their lifetime.

7. Alzheimer's Disease: Alzheimer's disease accounts for approximately 60-80% of all dementia cases.

8. Caregiver Statistics: More than 11 million family members and unpaid caregivers provided an estimated 18.4 billion hours of care to people with Alzheimer's or other dementias in the U.S. in 2023.

9. Economic Cost: The total cost of health care, long-term care, and hospice services for people age 65 and older with dementia is estimated at $360 billion in the U.S. for 2024.

10. Age Factor: The likelihood of developing dementia increases significantly with age; approximately 13.1% of individuals aged 85 and older have a dementia diagnosis.

11. Cognitive Decline: Dementia can lead to significant memory loss, impaired reasoning, and changes in behavior and personality.

12. Symptoms: Common symptoms include forgetfulness, difficulty communicating, confusion about time or place, and changes in mood or behavior.

13. Diagnosis: There is no single test for dementia; diagnosis typically involves a combination of medical history, cognitive tests, and brain imaging.

14. Risk Factors: Age, genetics, cardiovascular health, and

lifestyle choices (such as diet and exercise) are significant risk factors for developing dementia.

15. Gender Differences: Women are more likely than men to develop dementia; this may be due to longer life expectancy.

16. Cultural Impact: Dementia affects individuals from all cultural backgrounds, but awareness and understanding can vary significantly across communities.

17. Care Home Residents: It is estimated that around 70% of residents in care homes have dementia or severe memory problems.

18. Community Living: Approximately two-thirds of individuals with dementia live in the community rather than institutional settings.

19. Behavioral Changes: Individuals with dementia may experience changes such as agitation, aggression, or withdrawal from social interactions.

20. Sundowning Syndrome: Many individuals with dementia experience increased confusion or agitation during late afternoon or evening hours.

21. Support Needs: More than 1.6 million Australians are involved in caring for someone living with dementia.

22. Early Detection Importance: Early diagnosis allows for better planning and management of care needs for individuals with dementia.

23. Public Health Concern: Dementia is considered a major public health issue due to its impact on individuals, families, and healthcare systems.

24. Dementia Types: In addition to Alzheimer's disease, other types include vascular dementia, Lewy body dementia, and frontotemporal dementia.

25. Cognitive Reserve Theory: Engaging in mentally stimulating activities throughout life may build cognitive reserve that helps delay the onset of symptoms.

26. Nutrition's Role: Diets rich in fruits, vegetables, whole grains, and healthy fats (like the Mediterranean diet) may reduce the risk of cognitive decline.

27. Physical Activity Benefits: Regular physical exercise is associated with a lower risk of developing dementia and improved overall brain health.

28. Emotional Impact on Caregivers: Caregiving for someone with dementia can lead to significant emotional distress and increased risk for mental health issues among caregivers.

29. Technology Use: Innovations like telehealth services and wearable devices are increasingly being used to support individuals with dementia and their caregivers.

30. Community Resources: Many communities offer support groups and resources specifically designed for families affected by dementia.

31. Legal Considerations: Establishing advance directives and power of attorney is crucial for ensuring that an individual's wishes regarding care are respected.

32. Cultural Sensitivity: Understanding cultural beliefs about aging and illness is essential for providing effective care to diverse populations.

33. Impact on Families: Families often experience anticipatory grief as they navigate the progression of their loved one's condition.

34. End-of-Life Care Needs: Individuals with advanced dementia require specialized end-of-life care that focuses on comfort and quality of life.

35. Research Funding Gaps: Despite the growing prevalence of dementia, funding for research lags behind other diseases like cancer or heart disease.

36. Awareness Campaigns: Public awareness campaigns play a critical role in educating communities about dementia risk factors and available resources.

37. Social Engagement Importance: Maintaining social connections can help mitigate feelings of isolation and depression among individuals with dementia.

38. Caregiver Training Programs: Specialized training programs can equip caregivers with skills needed to manage challenging behaviors effectively.

39. Impact on Healthcare Systems: The increasing number of individuals living with dementia places significant strain on healthcare systems worldwide.

40. Multidisciplinary Approaches: Effective dementia care often involves a team approach that includes medical professionals, social workers, therapists, and family members.

41. Financial Burden on Families: The costs associated with caring for someone with dementia can be substantial, often leading to financial strain on families.

42. Stigma Reduction Efforts: Reducing stigma associated with dementia is essential for encouraging early diagnosis and improving access to care services.

43. Dementia-Friendly Communities: Initiatives aimed at creating supportive environments can enhance the quality of life for individuals living with dementia.

44. Research on Biomarkers: Ongoing research into biomarkers may lead to earlier diagnosis and better-targeted treatments for various forms of dementia.

45. Impact of COVID-19: The pandemic has exacerbated challenges faced by individuals living with dementia, including increased isolation and disruption of care services.

46. Supportive Housing Models: Innovative housing models designed specifically for individuals with dementia promote independence while ensuring safety and support.

47. Volunteer Opportunities: Many organizations rely on volunteers to provide companionship and support to individuals living with dementia in community settings.

48. Crisis Intervention Services: Access to crisis intervention services can help manage acute behavioral episodes effectively without resorting to hospitalization.

49. Family Dynamics Changes: The onset of a loved one's dementia can alter family roles and dynamics significantly as caregiving responsibilities shift.

50. Ongoing Education Needs: Continuous education about best practices in dementia care is vital for both professional caregivers and family members alike.

51. Genetic Factors: Certain genetic mutations, such as those associated with familial Alzheimer's disease, can significantly increase the risk of developing dementia.

52. Environmental Factors: Exposure to environmental toxins, such as heavy metals and air pollution, has been linked to an increased risk of cognitive decline and dementia.

53. Sleep Disorders: Sleep disturbances, including sleep apnea and insomnia, may contribute to cognitive decline and increase the risk of developing dementia.

54. Depression and Dementia: Depression is both a risk factor for and a symptom of dementia. Individuals with depression may experience cognitive impairment that can mimic dementia.

55. Cognitive Training Programs: Engaging in cognitive training programs has shown promise in improving specific cognitive functions and may help delay the onset of dementia symptoms.

56. Importance of Hydration: Dehydration can exacerbate confusion and cognitive decline in individuals with dementia, making proper hydration essential for maintaining cognitive function.

57. Art Therapy Benefits: Art therapy can provide a creative outlet for individuals with dementia, helping to improve mood, reduce anxiety, and enhance communication.

58. Music Therapy: Music therapy has been shown to evoke memories and emotions in individuals with dementia, fostering connections and improving overall well-being.

59. Dementia and Diabetes: There is a significant association between diabetes and an increased risk of developing dementia, particularly vascular dementia.

60. Social Isolation Risks: Social isolation is a significant risk factor for cognitive decline; maintaining social interactions can help protect against memory loss.

61. Importance of Routine: Establishing daily routines can provide structure and familiarity for individuals with dementia, reducing anxiety and confusion.

62. Nutritional Supplements: Some studies suggest that certain nutritional supplements, such as omega-3 fatty acids and antioxidants, may have protective effects on brain health.

63. Physical Therapy Benefits: Physical therapy can help individuals with dementia maintain mobility and independence while reducing the risk of falls.

64. Impact on Relationships: Dementia can strain relationships between individuals living with the condition and their family members due to changes in behavior and communication challenges.

65. Legal Rights: Individuals with dementia retain certain legal rights until they are deemed incapable of making decisions; understanding these rights is crucial for caregivers.

66. Crisis Planning: Developing a crisis plan can help families prepare for potential emergencies related to behavioral changes or health issues in individuals with dementia.

67. Technology-Assisted Care: Telehealth services have become increasingly important in providing care for individuals with dementia, especially during times of social distancing.

68. Dementia-Friendly Policies: Advocacy for policies that support individuals with dementia—such as accessible public spaces and transportation—can enhance quality of life.

69. Workplace Support: Employers are increasingly recognizing the need to support employees who are caregivers for family members with dementia through flexible work arrangements.

70. Cultural Competence in Care: Understanding cultural differences in perceptions of aging and illness is essential for providing effective care to diverse populations affected by dementia.

71. Family Meetings: Regular family meetings can facilitate communication among caregivers, helping to coordinate care strategies and share responsibilities effectively.

72. Holistic Approaches: Integrating holistic approaches—such as mindfulness, yoga, or meditation—can improve emotional well-being for both individuals with dementia and their caregivers.

73. Research on Loneliness: Studies indicate that loneliness can exacerbate cognitive decline; addressing social needs is crucial for maintaining mental health in individuals with dementia.

74. Dementia Simulations: Training programs that use simulation techniques to mimic the experiences of living with dementia can enhance empathy among caregivers and healthcare professionals.

75. Supportive Legislation: Legislative efforts aimed at improving funding for research and support services are critical for addressing the growing burden of dementia care on families and healthcare systems.

76. Community Awareness Programs: Initiatives aimed at educating the public about dementia can help reduce stigma and promote understanding within communities.

77. End-of-Life Planning Conversations: Encouraging open discussions about end-of-life preferences early in the disease process ensures that individuals' wishes are respected as their condition progresses.

CHAPTER 29: FUTURE TRENDS IN DEMENTIA CARE

As we look to the future, the landscape of dementia care is poised for transformation. Driven by advancements in research, technology, and innovative care models, the coming years hold promise for improving the quality of life for individuals living with dementia and their caregivers. This chapter explores emerging trends, ongoing research, and hopeful developments that are shaping the future of dementia care.

Advancements in Research and Treatments

Research into dementia has made significant strides, with a focus on developing new treatments and understanding the underlying mechanisms of the disease. Recent advancements include:

- New Drug Developments: For the first time in years, drug companies have approached regulatory bodies for approval of medications that may slow the progression of Alzheimer's disease. While some treatments have faced challenges regarding cost-effectiveness and accessibility, ongoing research continues to explore viable options (Alzheimer's Society, 2019).

- Gene Therapy Initiatives: Innovative gene therapy approaches are being explored to address inherited forms of dementia. The UK Dementia Research Institute is investing in initiatives aimed at correcting genetic mutations that contribute to neurodegenerative diseases (Alzheimer's Society, 2019).

- Lifestyle Interventions: Research indicates that adopting certain lifestyle choices—such as regular physical activity, a balanced diet, and social engagement—can reduce the risk of developing dementia. A study highlighted that these simple lifestyle modifications could potentially prevent up to 35% of dementia cases (Alzheimer's Society, 2019).

Enhanced Training for Caregivers

As the demand for dementia care rises, so does the need for enhanced training for caregivers. Recognition of caregiving as a skilled profession is growing, leading to:

- Specialized Training Programs: Many organizations are now offering advanced training beyond basic certification. This includes education on person-centered care approaches, communication techniques, and understanding behavioral changes associated with dementia (CPD Online).

- Continuous Professional Development: Encouraging ongoing education for caregivers ensures they remain informed about best practices and new developments in dementia care. This investment in training ultimately leads to improved outcomes for individuals with dementia (CPD Online).

Community-Based Support Models

Innovative community-based models are emerging as effective alternatives to traditional care settings. These models focus on creating supportive environments that prioritize quality of life:

- Dementia-Friendly Villages: Inspired by successful international examples like the Hogeweyk Dementia Village in the Netherlands, these communities are designed to resemble real towns where individuals can live independently while receiving necessary support. Research has shown that such environments can reduce feelings of loneliness and aggression while promoting cognitive engagement (CPD Online).

- Integrated Care Approaches: Multidisciplinary teams—including psychiatrists, occupational therapists, and social workers—are increasingly collaborating to address the diverse needs of individuals with dementia. This holistic approach ensures comprehensive care tailored to each person's unique circumstances (CPD Online).

Policy and Advocacy Efforts

Advocacy plays a crucial role in shaping policies that improve dementia care. Organizations like Alzheimer's Society are actively working to influence legislation and promote awareness:

- Funding for Research and Care: Advocates are calling for increased funding for dementia research and improved social care services. This includes efforts to standardize care across regions and ensure equitable access to resources (CPD Online).

- Public Awareness Campaigns: Raising awareness about risk factors, prevention strategies, and the importance of early diagnosis is essential for improving outcomes. Targeted campaigns aim to educate communities about dementia and reduce stigma surrounding the condition (CPD Online).

Hopes for Improved Quality of Life

The ultimate goal of advancements in dementia care is to enhance the quality of life for individuals living with the condition. Key hopes for the future include:

- Global Collaboration: Efforts to foster international partnerships among researchers, healthcare providers, and policymakers are crucial for addressing global challenges related to dementia care. Collaborative initiatives can lead to shared knowledge and resources that benefit individuals worldwide (CPD Online).

- Innovative Technologies: The integration of technology into daily care routines—such as telehealth services, wearable devices, and smart home technologies—holds promise for enhancing safety and independence for individuals with dementia (Alzheimer's Society, 2019).

Summary

The future of dementia care is bright with potential as research advances, caregiver training improves, community-based models emerge, and advocacy efforts gain momentum. By embracing these trends and innovations, we can create an environment that prioritizes dignity, independence, and quality of life for individuals living with dementia.

As Dr. David Knopman states: "The convergence of innovation in treatment and compassionate caregiving will define the next era of support for those affected by dementia." By fostering collaboration among stakeholders at all levels—researchers, caregivers, policymakers, and communities—we can work toward a future where individuals living with dementia receive the compassionate care they deserve while maintaining their dignity and autonomy.

CHAPTER 30: PERSONAL STORIES AND CASE STUDIES

Personal stories and case studies provide invaluable insights into the lived experiences of individuals with dementia and their caregivers. These narratives highlight the challenges faced, the coping strategies employed, and the profound moments of connection that can emerge despite the difficulties. This chapter shares several poignant examples that illustrate the diverse experiences within the dementia journey.

Case Study 1: Mary's Journey with Alzheimer's Disease

Mary, a 72-year-old retired teacher, was diagnosed with Alzheimer's disease three years ago. Initially, her family noticed subtle changes in her memory, such as forgetting names and misplacing items. As her condition progressed, she began to experience confusion about time and place.

To support Mary, her family implemented a structured daily routine that included familiar activities like reading and gardening. They also engaged her in reminiscence therapy by looking through old photo albums and discussing significant life events. Mary's daughter remarked, "These moments of connection remind us of who she is beneath the diagnosis; they bring joy to our days."

Research supports the effectiveness of structured routines and reminiscence therapy in enhancing quality of life for individuals with dementia (Simmons-Stern et al., 2010). Mary's story exemplifies how tailored interventions can foster meaningful engagement and emotional well-being.

Case Study 2: John and His Caregiver

John, a 68-year-old man living with vascular dementia, exhibited significant behavioral changes, including agitation and wandering. His spouse, Linda, faced considerable stress managing these behaviors while maintaining her own well-being.

Linda sought support through a local caregiver support group, where she learned valuable strategies for managing John's agitation. By identifying triggers—such as loud noises or unfamiliar environments—Linda was able to create a calmer home atmosphere. She also implemented redirection techniques during moments of frustration.

"Joining the support group was a turning point for me," Linda shared. "I realized I wasn't alone in this journey; we all face similar challenges."

Studies indicate that caregiver support groups can significantly reduce stress and improve coping strategies (Kramer et al., 2014), underscoring the importance of community in navigating dementia care.

Case Study 3: The Impact of Technology on Care

The Smith family integrated technology into their care approach for their father, who has late-stage Alzheimer's disease. They utilized a wearable device that monitored his location and activity levels, providing peace of mind while allowing him to maintain some independence.

The device alerted family members when he wandered beyond a designated area, enabling them to intervene quickly if necessary. "It felt liberating to know we could keep him safe without hovering over him all day," his daughter noted.

This case highlights how technological innovations can enhance safety and independence for individuals with dementia while alleviating caregiver anxiety (Alzheimer's Society, 2019).

Case Study 4: Community-Based Support in Action

Inspired by successful models like the Hogeweyk Dementia Village in the Netherlands, a community in Warwick, England, developed a purpose-built facility designed to resemble a mini-town where individuals with dementia can live independently while receiving necessary support.

Residents benefit from higher-than-average ratios of caregivers to patients and engage in daily activities that promote socialization and cognitive engagement. Research shows that such environments can reduce levels of loneliness, aggression, and depression in dementia patients while slowing cognitive decline (CPD Online).

One resident's family member remarked, "Seeing my mother thrive in this environment has been heartwarming. She feels at home here."

Summary

These personal stories and case studies illustrate the diverse experiences of those affected by dementia. They emphasize the importance of tailored interventions—whether through structured routines, community support, or technology—in enhancing quality of life for individuals with dementia and their caregivers. Through these experiences, we can foster understanding and empathy within society while inspiring others facing similar challenges to seek support and embrace innovative solutions.

Together, we can reclaim memories, nurture relationships, and create a supportive environment that celebrates life in all its complexities.

CHAPTER 31: HOPES FOR THE FUTURE OF DEMENTIA CARE

As we look toward the future, the landscape of dementia care is evolving rapidly, driven by advancements in research, technology, and innovative care models. This chapter explores the hopes and expectations for the future of dementia care, focusing on improved quality of life for individuals living with dementia, enhanced caregiver training, community-based support models, and ongoing advocacy efforts.

Advancements in Research and Treatments

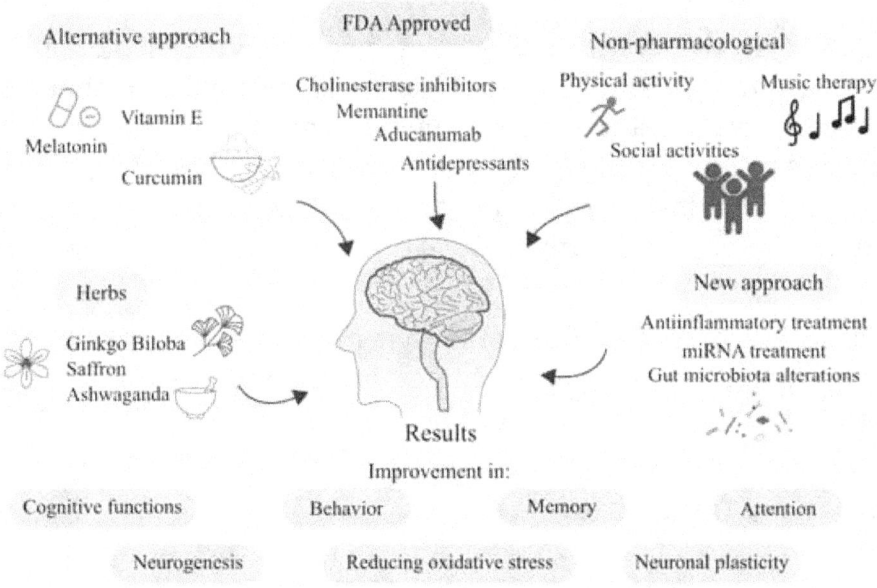

New and alternative approach to treatment of AD

The quest for effective treatments for dementia has gained momentum in recent years. While no cure currently exists, significant progress is being made in understanding the disease and developing potential therapies. For instance, recent research has highlighted promising developments such as:

- **New Drug Approvals**: In 2023, a groundbreaking drug was licensed to treat mild cognitive impairment associated with Alzheimer's disease. Although its high cost has raised concerns about accessibility, it represents a significant step forward in drug development (CPD Online).

- **Gene Therapy Initiatives**: Innovative approaches are being explored to address inherited forms of dementia through gene therapy. The UK Dementia Research Institute is investing in initiatives aimed at correcting genetic mutations that contribute to neurodegenerative diseases (Alzheimer's Society).

- **Lifestyle Interventions:** Studies have shown that adopting healthy lifestyle choices—such as regular physical activity, a balanced diet, and social engagement—can significantly reduce the risk of developing dementia. The Alzheimer's Society states that simple lifestyle modifications could prevent up to 35% of dementia cases (Alzheimer's Society).

These advancements fuel hope that more effective treatments will emerge, improving outcomes for individuals living with dementia.

Enhanced Training for Caregivers

As the demand for dementia care increases, so does the need for enhanced training for caregivers. Recognizing caregiving as a skilled profession is essential for providing quality care. Key developments in caregiver training include:

- Specialized Training Programs: Many organizations are now offering advanced training beyond basic certification. This includes education on person-centered care approaches, communication techniques, and understanding behavioral changes associated with dementia (CPD Online).

- Continuous Professional Development: Encouraging ongoing education for caregivers ensures they remain informed about best practices and new developments in dementia care. This investment in training ultimately leads to improved outcomes for individuals with dementia (CPD Online).

Research indicates that well-trained caregivers can significantly enhance the quality of life for individuals living with dementia by providing compassionate and informed support (Kramer et al., 2014).

Community-Based Support Models

Innovative community-based models are emerging as effective alternatives to traditional care settings. These models focus on creating supportive environments that prioritize quality of life:

- Dementia-Friendly Villages: Inspired by successful international examples like the Hogeweyk Dementia Village in the Netherlands, communities are developing purpose-built facilities designed to resemble real towns where individuals can live independently while receiving necessary support. Research shows that such environments can reduce levels of loneliness and aggression while promoting cognitive engagement (CPD Online).

- Integrated Care Approaches: Multidisciplinary teams—including psychiatrists, occupational therapists, and social workers—are increasingly collaborating to address the diverse needs of individuals with dementia. This holistic approach ensures comprehensive care tailored to each person's unique circumstances (CPD Online).

The hope is that these community-based models will become more widespread, providing individuals with dementia opportunities to thrive in supportive environments.

Policy and Advocacy Efforts

Advocacy plays a crucial role in shaping policies that improve dementia care. Organizations like Alzheimer's Society are actively working to influence legislation and promote awareness:

- Funding for Research and Care: Advocates are calling for increased funding for dementia research and improved social care services. This includes efforts to standardize care across regions and ensure equitable access to resources (CPD Online).

- Public Awareness Campaigns: Raising awareness about risk factors, prevention strategies, and the importance of early diagnosis is essential for improving outcomes. Targeted campaigns aim to educate communities about dementia and reduce stigma surrounding the condition (CPD Online).

The hope is that increased advocacy will lead to better social care systems that prioritize the needs of individuals living with dementia.

Summary

The future of dementia care holds immense promise as advancements in research, caregiver training, community-based support models, and advocacy efforts converge to improve the quality of life for those affected by this condition. As Dr. David Knopman emphasizes: "The convergence of innovation in treatment and compassionate caregiving will define the next era of support for those affected by dementia."

By fostering collaboration among stakeholders at all levels —researchers, caregivers, policymakers, and communities—we can work toward a future where individuals living with dementia receive the compassionate care they deserve while maintaining their dignity and autonomy.

As we continue this journey together, let us remain hopeful and committed to creating a world where every individual living with dementia can thrive amidst the challenges they face.

CHAPTER 32: CURRENT RESEARCH AND FUTURE DIRECTIONS IN TREATMENT

The landscape of Alzheimer's disease (AD) treatment is evolving rapidly, driven by advances in research and a deeper understanding of the disease's underlying mechanisms. This chapter reviews current research initiatives, promising drug candidates, and future directions in the treatment of dementia, emphasizing the potential for disease-modifying therapies.

Promising Drug Candidates

Lecanemab

Lecanemab, recently approved by the FDA, represents a significant advancement in AD treatment. This monoclonal antibody targets amyloid-beta (Aβ) protofibrils, aiming to reduce amyloid plaque levels in the brain. In clinical trials, lecanemab demonstrated a 27% slowing of cognitive decline over 18 months compared to placebo groups (van Dyck et al., 2023) . Dr. Christopher van Dyck noted, "This is the first treatment in our history that shows an unequivocal slowing of decline in Alzheimer's disease" (Yale Medicine) .

Donanemab

Another promising candidate is donanemab, which targets Aβ plaques and has shown up to a 60% slowing of cognitive decline when administered early in the disease course (BrightFocus Foundation) . The TRAILBLAZER-ALZ trials have demonstrated that donanemab not only reduces amyloid burden but also improves daily functioning in patients. As reported, "The drug appeared to slow how fast memory and thinking get worse by 20-60%, depending on the memory test used" (Alzheimer's Society) .

Blarcamesine

Blarcamesine is noteworthy for its dual action: it targets both amyloid and tau proteins, potentially addressing multiple aspects of AD pathology. Recent trials indicated that participants experienced over a 25% slowing of cognitive decline (Nature Reviews) . This broad-spectrum approach may offer a more comprehensive treatment strategy for AD.

Immunotherapy Approaches

Immunotherapy is emerging as a promising avenue for AD treatment. By harnessing the immune system to target pathological proteins, researchers aim to halt or reverse neurodegeneration. Various strategies include:

- Monoclonal Antibodies: Drugs like lecanemab and donanemab fall into this category, targeting Aβ accumulation directly.

- Vaccines: Experimental vaccines aim to stimulate an immune response against Aβ or tau proteins. While results have been mixed, ongoing trials continue to explore their potential.

According to a report from the NHS, "Some monoclonal antibody medicines have shown promising results and are now being considered as treatments for Alzheimer's" (NHS).

Gene-Based Therapies

Gene-based therapies are gaining traction as researchers explore ways to modify genetic risk factors associated with dementia. These therapies aim to reduce the production of harmful proteins or enhance neuronal resilience. For example, targeting genes linked to tau pathology could provide new avenues for intervention.

Repurposing Existing Medications

Repurposing existing drugs offers a faster route to potential AD treatments. Medications originally developed for other conditions—such as diabetes or hypertension—are being investigated for their effects on cognitive function. This approach could expedite the availability of effective therapies while minimizing development costs.

Future Directions

The future of AD treatment lies in personalized medicine —tailoring interventions based on individual genetic profiles and biomarker assessments. Ongoing research aims to identify specific patient populations that may benefit most from targeted therapies.

Moreover, early intervention remains crucial. As Dr. van Dyck emphasizes, "We may see a larger benefit if we intervene before significant brain damage has occurred" (Yale Medicine) . The AHEAD study is currently exploring this concept by enrolling cognitively normal individuals at high risk for AD.

Summary

The field of Alzheimer's disease treatment is witnessing unprecedented advancements, with several promising drug candidates on the horizon and innovative therapeutic approaches being explored. While challenges remain, ongoing research offers hope for more effective interventions that can modify disease progression and improve quality of life for those affected by dementia.

"The next generation of treatments is making its way through clinical trials... with many promising developments expected in the near future" (BrightFocus Foundation).

CHAPTER 33: CONCLUSION AND CALL TO ACTION

As we conclude *Reclaiming Memories: A Guide to Preventing and Navigating Dementia*, it is essential to reflect on the journey we have taken through the complexities of dementia care. From understanding the condition and its emotional impacts to exploring effective communication techniques, daily living strategies, and future trends, this book has aimed to equip readers with knowledge and tools to navigate the challenges posed by dementia.

Recap of Key Insights

Throughout this book, we have emphasized several key insights:

1. Understanding Dementia, A biochemical perspective: Recognizing the various types of dementia and their symptoms through the lens of Biochemistry is crucial for early detection and effective management. The importance of education cannot be overstated, as knowledge empowers families and caregivers to respond appropriately to the needs of individuals with dementia.

2. Emotional Impact: The emotional toll of dementia affects not only those diagnosed but also their families and caregivers. Strategies for managing these emotions—through open communication, support groups, and self-care—are vital for fostering resilience.

3. Effective Communication: Utilizing simple language, maintaining eye contact, and employing non-verbal cues can significantly improve interactions with individuals living with dementia. These techniques help bridge the gap created by cognitive decline.

4. Daily Living Strategies: Creating a safe environment, engaging in meaningful activities, and establishing routines promote independence and enhance quality of life for individuals with dementia.

5. Managing Behavioral Changes: Understanding the underlying causes of behavioral changes allows caregivers to implement effective strategies that address agitation, wandering, and other challenging behaviors.

6. Legal and Financial Considerations: Advance care planning, establishing power of attorney, and proactive financial management are critical components of ensuring that individuals with dementia receive appropriate care aligned with their wishes.

7. Future Trends: The landscape of dementia care is evolving, with advancements in research, caregiver training, community-based models, and advocacy efforts paving the way for improved outcomes.

A Vision for the Future

The future holds promise for individuals living with dementia and their caregivers. As highlighted in recent research and developments:

- Innovative Treatments: Ongoing research into new drugs and therapies offers hope for slowing disease progression. The recent approval of drugs targeting cognitive impairment associated with Alzheimer's disease marks a significant step forward (Alzheimer's Society).

- Community-Based Support Models: The emergence of dementia-friendly communities—such as purpose-built facilities designed to resemble real towns—demonstrates a commitment to enhancing quality of life through person-centered care (CPD Online).

- Advocacy Efforts: Organizations like Alzheimer's Society are tirelessly working to influence policy changes that improve the quality of life for people living with dementia. Increased funding for research and better social care are essential components of this advocacy (CPD Online).

Call to Action

As we move forward, it is imperative that we all take action:

1. Educate yourself and others: Knowledge is power. Share what you have learned about dementia with family members, friends, and your community. Raising awareness can help reduce stigma and foster understanding.

2. Support Research Initiatives: Consider supporting organizations dedicated to dementia research through donations or participation in fundraising events. Every contribution helps advance our understanding of this complex condition.

3. Advocate for Change: Engage in advocacy efforts at local and national levels. Support policies that prioritize funding for dementia care, research initiatives, and community resources.

4. Foster Community Connections: Encourage your community to become more dementia-friendly by promoting inclusive practices that support individuals living with dementia and their families.

5. Take Care of Yourself: If you are a caregiver, prioritize your well-being by seeking support through local groups or online forums. Remember that caring for yourself enables you to provide better care for others.

Conclusion

In closing, *Reclaiming Memories* is not just a guide; it is a call to action for all of us, Individuals,—families, caregivers, healthcare professionals, researchers, and advocates—to work together in creating a world where this menace is checked/prevented through awareness, and individuals living with dementia can thrive amidst the challenges they face. By embracing compassion, understanding, and innovation, we can *reclaim memories*, nurture connections, and foster hope for a brighter future in dementia care.

GLOSSARY OF TERMS

A

Acetylcholine: A neurotransmitter that is involved in muscle contraction, learning, and memory.
Adenosine triphosphate (ATP): The molecule that cells use for energy.
Agnosia: The inability to recognize familiar objects, people, or sounds despite having intact sensory function. This can affect communication and daily living.

Alzheimer's Disease (AD): The most common form of dementia, characterized by progressive cognitive decline, memory loss, and behavioral changes, often associated with amyloid plaques and tau tangles in the brain.

Amyloid beta protein: A protein fragment that forms plaques in the brains of people with Alzheimer's disease.
Amyloid plaques: Clumps of beta-amyloid protein that form in the brains of people with Alzheimer's disease.
Antioxidants: Substances that can neutralize free radicals, which are highly reactive molecules that can damage cells.

Apathy: A lack of interest or emotional response, which can be mistaken for depression. It often manifests as a diminished motivation to engage in activities.

Apolipoprotein E (ApoE): A protein involved in lipid metabolism that has been linked to Alzheimer's disease risk, particularly the ApoE4 variant, which increases susceptibility to the disease.

Apraxia: The loss of the ability to perform purposeful movements or tasks, such as dressing or using utensils, despite having the physical capability to do so.

Astrocytes: Star-shaped cells in the brain that support neurons and help to maintain the blood-brain barrier.

Axon: A long, slender projection from a neuron that sends signals to other neurons.

B

Behavioral Neurologist: A medical doctor who specializes in diagnosing and treating memory disorders and behavioral changes associated with neurological conditions.

Beta-Amyloid: A protein that accumulates in the brains of individuals with Alzheimer's disease, forming plaques that disrupt cell function.

Biochemical Mechanisms: The chemical processes and interactions at the molecular level that contribute to biological functions and disease states.

Brain-derived neurotrophic factor (BDNF): A protein that is important for brain health. It promotes the growth and survival of neurons and synapses.

C

Cognition: The mental processes involved in acquiring knowledge and understanding through thought, experience, and the senses. This includes memory, attention, and problem-solving.

Cognitive Decline: A gradual deterioration in cognitive abilities, including memory, reasoning, and problem-solving skills, often observed in dementia.

Cognitive Stimulation Therapy (CST): A structured program designed to improve cognitive function through engaging activities and discussions in a group setting.

D

Delusion: A persistent belief that is contradicted by reality or rational argument. Individuals with dementia may experience delusions as part of their condition.

Dementia: An umbrella term for a range of symptoms that result from various diseases affecting the brain, leading to a decline in cognitive function, memory, and the ability to perform daily activities.
Dendrites: Short, branching extensions from a neuron that receive signals from other neurons.

Dopamine: A neurotransmitter that is involved in reward, pleasure, and motivation.

Durable Power of Attorney (DPOA): A legal document that allows an individual to appoint someone else to make healthcare or financial decisions on their behalf if they become incapacitated.

E

Early Stage Dementia: The initial phase of dementia where symptoms are mild but may include memory loss and difficulty with complex tasks.

End-of-Life Care: Support and medical care provided during the final phase of life, focusing on comfort and quality of life for individuals with terminal conditions.

Excitotoxicity: The process by which excessive stimulation of neurons by neurotransmitters, particularly glutamate, leads to neuronal injury and death.

F

Free radicals: Highly reactive molecules that can damage cells.

Frontotemporal dementia (FTD): A neurodegenerative disease that affects the frontal and temporal lobes of the brain.

G

GABA: An inhibitory neurotransmitter that is involved in relaxation and sleep.

Glutamate: An excitatory neurotransmitter that is involved in learning and memory.

Glycolysis: The first stage of cellular respiration, in which glucose is broken down into pyruvate.

H

Hippocampus: A region of the brain crucial for memory

formation. It is often affected early in Alzheimer's disease.

K

Krebs cycle: The second stage of cellular respiration, in which pyruvate is broken down into carbon dioxide and hydrogen ions.

L

Lewy Body Dementia: A type of dementia characterized by abnormal protein deposits (Lewy bodies) in the brain, leading to cognitive fluctuations, visual hallucinations, and motor symptoms similar to Parkinson's disease.

Long-Term Memory: The storage system for information retained over extended periods. Individuals with dementia may struggle with retrieving long-term memories.

M

Microtubules: Long, thin protein filaments that help to give cells their shape and structure.

Mild Cognitive Impairment (MCI): A condition characterized by noticeable memory problems greater than expected for a person's age but not severe enough to interfere significantly with daily life. MCI can be a precursor to dementia.

Mitochondria: The "powerhouses" of the cell. They are responsible for producing energy in the form of ATP.

N

Neurodegeneration: The progressive loss of structure or function of neurons, leading to conditions such as Alzheimer's disease and other forms of dementia.

Neurofibrillary tangles: Twisted filaments of tau protein that form in the brains of people with Alzheimer's disease.

Neuron: A nerve cell.

Neurotransmitters: Chemical messengers that transmit signals between neurons; key neurotransmitters involved in dementia include acetylcholine, glutamate, dopamine, and norepinephrine.

Norepinephrine: A neurotransmitter that is involved in the fight-or-flight response.

O

Oxidative Stress: An imbalance between free radicals and antioxidants in the body, leading to cellular damage; implicated in neurodegenerative diseases like Alzheimer's.

P

Palliative Care: Specialized medical care focused on providing relief from symptoms and stress associated with serious illnesses. It aims to improve quality of life for both patients and families.

Parkinson's disease: A neurodegenerative disease that affects movement. It is characterized by the death of dopamine-producing neurons in the substantia nigra.

Person-Centered Care: An approach that prioritizes the individual's preferences, needs, and values in all aspects of care, fostering dignity and respect.

Protein Misfolding: The process by which proteins fail to fold into their correct three-dimensional shapes, leading to dysfunctional proteins that can aggregate and cause disease.

R

Reminiscence Therapy: A therapeutic approach that encourages individuals with dementia to recall past experiences using prompts such as photographs or music, helping to stimulate memory and emotional connection.

S

Serotonin: A neurotransmitter that is involved in mood, appetite, and sleep.

Sundowning: A phenomenon where individuals with dementia experience increased confusion or agitation during the late afternoon or evening hours.

Synapse: The junction between two neurons.

T

Telehealth: The use of digital information and communication technologies to access healthcare services remotely. Telehealth can provide support for individuals with dementia who may have difficulty traveling to appointments.

Tau Protein: A protein associated with microtubule stability in neurons; hyperphosphorylated tau is a key feature of neurofibrillary tangles found in Alzheimer's disease.

V

Vascular Dementia: A type of dementia caused by reduced blood flow to the brain due to strokes or other vascular conditions, leading to cognitive decline.

BIBLIOGRAPHY

Books

1. Alzheimer's Society. (2019). Dementia: The One Stop Guide. London: Alzheimer's Society.

2. Agronin, M. (2017). The Dementia Caregiver: A Guide to Caring for Someone with Alzheimer's Disease and Other Neurocognitive Disorders. New York: Oxford University Press.

3. Andrews, J. (2014). Dementia: The One Stop Guide. London: Penguin Books.

4. Brooker, D., Bruce, M., & Lillyman, S. (2022). Care Fit for VIPS: A Pocket Guide to Person-Centred Care for People with Dementia. Jessica Kingsley Publishers.

5. James, O. (2009). Contented Dementia: 24-Hour Wraparound Care for Lifelong Wellbeing. London: Vermilion.

6. Kitwood, T., & Brooker, D. (2022). Dementia Reconsidered Revisited: The Person Comes First. Jessica Kingsley Publishers.

7. Knopman, D. S., & Jones, D. T. (2021). Alzheimer Disease and Dementia: A Comprehensive Guide for Patients and Families. New York: Oxford University Press.

8. Mace, N. L., & Rabins, P. V. (2016). The 36-Hour Day: A Family Guide to Caring for People Who Have Alzheimer Disease, Related Dementias, and Memory Loss. Baltimore: Johns Hopkins University Press.

9. Power, G. A. (2010). Dementia Beyond Disease: Enhancing Well-Being. Baltimore: Health Professions Press.

10. Wiles, N. J. (2020). Alzheimer's Care: The Caregiver's Guide to Understanding Alzheimer's Disease & Best Practices to Care for People with Alzheimer's & Dementia. New York: CreateSpace Independent Publishing Platform.

11. Whitworth, H., & Whitworth, J. (2018). A Caregiver's Guide to Lewy Body Dementia. New York: Health Professions Press.

12. Weatherill, G. (2018). The Caregiver's Guide to Dementia: Practical Advice for Caring for Yourself and Your Loved One. New York: Health Professions Press.

Articles and Reports

1. BMC Geriatrics. (2018). "Improving End-of-Life Care in Patients with Dementia." Retrieved from [BMC Geriatrics] (https://bmcgeriatr.biomedcentral.com/articles/1 0.1186/s12877-018-0797-2).

2. Budin-Ljøsne, I., et al. (2022). "Public perceptions of dementia and mental health: a nationwide survey." BMC Public Health, 22(1), 1234.

3. Cummings, J., Aisen, P., Bateman, R., et al. (2022). "Alzheimer's disease drug development pipeline: 2022." Nature Reviews Drug Discovery, 21(5), 307-308.

4. Dening, T., et al. (2013). "Advance Care Planning in Dementia." International Journal of Geriatric Psychiatry, 28(1), 1-7.

5. Gitlin, L.N., et al. (2006). "Caregiver Intervention Research in Dementia Care: A Review of the Evidence." Journal of the American Geriatrics Society, 54(12), 1919-1924.

6. Griciuc, A., & Tanzi, R.E. (2021). "Genetics of Alzheimer's disease." Nature Reviews Genetics, 22(3), 163-177.

7. Kessing, L.V., et al. (2010). "The Impact of Depression on Cognitive Functioning in Older Adults." Journal of Affective Disorders, 125(1-3), 1-12.

8. Knapp, M., et al. (2006). "Cognitive stimulation therapy for dementia: a systematic review." Age and Ageing, 35(6), 602-608.

9. Kramer, A., et al. (2014). "Caregiver Stress and Its Impact on Quality of Life." American Journal of Nursing, 114(12), 34-42.

10. Livingston, G., et al. (2017). "Dementia prevention, intervention, and care." The Lancet, 390(10113), 2673-2734.

11. Livingston, G., et al. (2020). "Dementia Prevention, Intervention, and Care." Lancet, 396(10248), 413-446.

12. Mather, M., et al. (2023). "The role of norepinephrine in cognitive aging." Psychological Bulletin, 149(1), 22-36.

13. Ngandu, T., et al. (2015). "A 2-year multidomain

intervention to prevent cognitive decline in at-risk elderly people: a randomized controlled trial." The Lancet, 385(9984), 2255-2263.

14. Simmons-Stern, N.R., et al. (2010). "The Effects of Reminiscence Therapy on Individuals with Dementia." Journal of Clinical Psychology, 66(11), 1155-1162.

15. Sofi, F., et al. (2010). "Adherence to Mediterranean diet and health status: meta-analysis." BMJ, 340, c1240.

16. van Dyck, C.H., Swanson, C.J., Aisen, P., et al. (2023). "Lecanemab in Early Alzheimer's Disease." New England Journal of Medicine, 388(1), 11-22.

17. World Health Organization (WHO). (2021). "Dementia Fact Sheet." Retrieved from [WHO](https://www.who.int/news-room/fact-sheets/detail/dementia).

18. Xie, L., et al. (2019). "Sleep drives metabolite clearance from the adult brain." Science, 363(6420), 880-884.

Online Resources

1. Alzheimer's Association. (2021). "Understanding Alzheimer's and Dementia." Retrieved from [Alzheimer's Association] (https://www.alz.org).

2. BrightFocus Foundation. "Alzheimer's Disease Research:

Current Trends and Future Directions." Retrieved from https://www.brightfocus.org/alzheimers/research.

3. Mayo Clinic: https://www.mayoclinic.org/

4. National Institute on Aging (NIA). "What Is Dementia?" Retrieved from [NIA](https://www.nia.nih.gov/health/what-dementia).

5. National Institutes of Health: https://www.nih.gov/

6. CPD Online Learning Resources on Dementia Care Training Programs.

7. World Health Organization: https://www.who.int/about

www.ingramcontent.com/pod-product-compliance
Lightning Source LLC
Chambersburg PA
CBHW071026240526
45469CB00006BD/2107